50 Ways to Prevent Colon Cancer

Other books by M. Sara Rosenthal:

The Thyroid Sourcebook
The Gynecological Sourcebook
The Pregnancy Sourcebook
The Fertility Sourcebook
The Breastfeeding Sourcebook
The Breast Sourcebook
The Gastrointestinal Sourcebook
Managing Your Diabetes
Managing Diabetes for Women
The Type 2 Diabetic Woman
The Thyroid Sourcebook for Women
Women & Depression
Women and Sadness: A Sane Approach to Depression
Women of the '60s Turning 50

50 Ways

to Prevent
Colon Cancer

M. Sara Rosenthal

Foreword by
Wm. Warren H. Rudd, M.D.,
F.R.C.S.(C.), F.A.C.S., author of
Advice from the Rudd Clinic:
A Guide to Colorectal Health

LOWELL HOUSE

LOS ANGELES

NTC/Contemporary Publishing Group

The purpose of this book is to educate. It is sold with the understanding that the publisher and author shall have neither liability nor responsibility for any injury caused or alleged to be caused directly or indirectly by the information contained in this book. While every effort has been made to ensure its accuracy, the book's contents should not be construed as medical advice. Each person's health needs are unique. To obtain recommendations appropriate to your particular situation, please consult a qualified health care provider.

Library of Congress Cataloging-in-Publication Data
Rosenthal, M. Sara.
    50 ways to prevent colon cancer / M. Sara Rosenthal.
        p. cm.
    Includes bibliographical references and index.
    ISBN 0-7373-0459-6
        1. Colon (Anatomy)—Cancer—Prevention. I. Title: Fifty ways to
        prevent colon cancer.
    II. Title.

RC280.C6 R67 2000
616.99'4347052—dc21   00-035216

Published by Lowell House
A division of NTC/Contemporary Publishing Group, Inc.
4255 West Touhy Avenue, Lincolnwood, Illinois 60646-1975 U.S.A.

Illustration on page xv by Elizabeth Weadon Massari
Illustrations on pages 28, 64, and 65 by Ilene Robinette
Interior design: Jack Lanning

Printed in the United States of America
International Standard Book Number: 0-7373-0459-6
00 01 02 03 04 ML 18 17 16 15 14 13 12 11 10 9 8 7 6 5 4 3 2 1

Contents

Foreword

If you've picked up this book, you probably have some concerns about colon cancer. Maybe you have a family member who has suffered from this disease, or maybe you've just had a birthday, and have heard or read that colon cancer is common in people over the age of forty-five. Whatever your reasons for picking up *50 Ways to Prevent Colon Cancer,* as a surgeon specializing in diseases of the colon and rectum, my advice is that you *read this book,* and then pass it on to friends and family members you care about.

Colon cancer is now the second most common "killer cancer" in both sexes—but it is almost entirely *preventable* if you have the right information. And if you're holding this book, you do!

This easy-to-read, informative, and comprehensive book will teach you things about colon cancer prevention that your own doctor may not even know. For instance, how many people really understand that almost all colon cancer can be caught early and treated, before it becomes life threatening, through appropriate, routine screening based on age rather than family history? Better still, how many know it can be stopped before it starts? How many people really understand how detrimental chronic constipation can be to your health and that to truly make a high-fiber diet work, you need to know that there are two kinds of fiber and that fiber needs to be combined with water in order to work its "magic"? How many people know the vitamins, foods, and herbs that can help combat colon and other cancers? Or how important physical activity is to lowering your risk of colon cancer? These are among the dozens of life-giving facts in this book.

The real tragedy of colon cancer is the absence of good information about how it can be prevented. That's why *50 Ways to Prevent Colon Cancer* is such an important book, and why I like recommending it to my patients. I'm delighted to light the path that shows you the ways to colon cancer prevention. By holding this in your hands, you're letting in the light.

—WM. WARREN H. RUDD, M.D., F.R.C.S.(C.),
F.A.C.S., Fellow, A.S.C.R.S.

Founder and Director, the Rudd Clinic
for Diseases of the Colon and Rectum,
Toronto, Canada,
Author of *Advice from the Rudd Clinic:
A Guide to Colorectal Health*, 2d ed.
(www.ruddclinic.com)

Acknowledgments

I wish to thank the following people, whose expertise and dedication helped to lay so much of the groundwork for this book:

Wm. Warren Rudd, M.D., F.R.C.S.(C.), F.A.C.S., Fellow, A.S.C.R.S., colon and rectal surgeon and founder and director of the Rudd Clinic for Diseases of the Colon and Rectum (Toronto), who is also the author of *Advice from the Rudd Clinic: A Guide to Colorectal Health*, served as medical advisor for this book. Dr. Rudd is a pioneer in his field; he endured harsh criticism from his peers and colleagues when he dared to open a clinic in 1969 dedicated to early detection and prevention of colon cancer. Today, Dr. Rudd's conviction that colon cancer is 90 percent preventable through early detection and removal of polyps—the precursors of colon cancer—is shared by all in his field. I was lucky to find his support for this work. Without his suggestions and contributions, this book would not have come to fruition.

A number of past medical advisors on previous works helped me to shape the content for this work. And so I wish to thank the following people (listed alphabetically): Gillian Arsenault, M.D., C.C.F.P., I.B.L.C., F.R.C.P.; Pamela Craig, M.D., F.A.C.S., Ph.D.; Masood Kahthamee, M.D., F.A.C.O.G.; Gary May, M.D., F.R.C.P.; James McSherry, M.B., Ch.B., F.C.F.P., F.R.C.G.P., F.A.A.F.P., F.A.B.M.P.; Suzanne Pratt, M.D., FA.C.O.G.; and Robert Volpe, M.D., F.R.C.P., F.A.C.P.

William Harvey, Ph.D., L.L.B., University of Toronto Joint Centre for Bioethics, whose devotion to bioethics has inspired me, continues to support my work, and makes it possible for me to have the courage to question and challenge issues in health care and medical ethics. Irving Rootman, Ph.D., Director, University of Toronto Centre for Health Promotion, continues to encourage my interest in primary prevention and health promotion issues.

Larissa Kostoff, my editorial consultant, worked very hard to make this book a reality. And finally, Hudson Perigo, my editor, made many wonderful and thoughtful suggestions to help make this book what it is.

Introduction

Yes, You Can Prevent Colon Cancer

Colorectal cancer (cancer in the colon and/or rectum) accounts for roughly 13 percent of all cancers, and is considered the second leading cause of cancer deaths, next to lung cancer. Colorectal cancer develops from an earlier, benign growth, known as a polyp (and in the plural, known as polyps). If you learn nothing else from this book, you'll receive "gold" if you remember this one sentence: *ALL colon cancer comes from polyps, but not all polyps become colon cancer.* What this means is that by screening for polyps on a regular basis, you can "catch" colon cancer before it ever develops. Think of polyp screening—or polyp hunting, as I call it—as the "Pap test" for colon cancer. In the same way that most women will be spared a diagnosis of cervical cancer, thanks to the Pap test, most people who go for regular polyp screening should be spared a diagnosis of colon cancer. Even if you are diagnosed with colorectal cancer, it's important to keep in mind that colorectal cancers develop in glandular tissue but are considered very curable when caught in an early stage.

If you can glean a second message from this book, remember this: *Colon cancer may be preventable through diet.* Of all the studies done on cancer and dietary fat, the strongest connections can be made between high-fat diets and colon cancer. In other words, people who consume large quantities of fat have higher rates of colon cancer. People who consume small quantities of fat have lower rates of colon cancer.

As for fiber, studies show that people who consume large quantities of fiber have lower rates of colon cancer, while people who consume small quantities of fiber have higher rates of colon cancer. In addition, people whose bowels are regular have a lower incidence of colon cancer than people who are chronically constipated. The third vital message of this book: *Drink water with fiber.* (See the Fiber section for more details.)

Studies also show that the number of calories in your diet—regardless of whether they're fat or fiber—can also increase the risk of colon cancer. One study found that in people under sixty-seven years old, an extra 500 calories a day can increase colon cancer risk in men by 15 percent and in women by 11 percent.

By lowering fat and increasing fiber, you'll greatly reduce your risk of colon cancer. The amazing thing is that no cancer expert will dispute this, even though they *can* dispute the fat-fiber connection when it comes to other cancers, such as breast. In fact, experts muse that by simply following the low-fat/high-fiber diet, you may be able to avoid 90 percent of all stomach and colon cancers and 20 percent of gallbladder, pancreas, mouth, pharynx, and esophageal cancers. Diet may even play a role in preventing lung cancer; recent studies show that people with low intakes of carotene

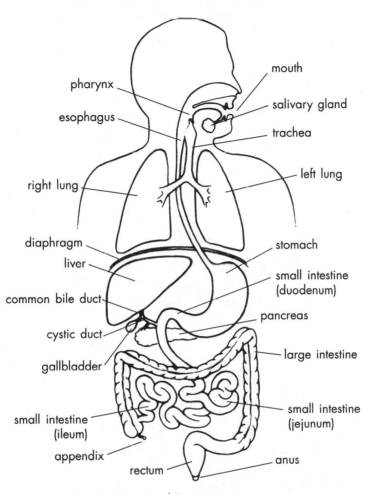

FIGURE 1 The Gastrointestinal Tract

(orange, red, and purple plant foods) have higher rates of lung cancer.

Finally, before you begin counting the ways you can prevent colon cancer, here's a diagram of your gastrointestinal tract. I guess you ought to know where your colon is, before I begin showing you fifty ways to prevent cancer there!

Screening for Colon Cancer

1. Understand the Purpose of Screening

The purpose of screening for colon cancer is to hunt down colon cancer "seedlings" known as polyps. Polyps are benign growths that can develop into colon cancer. All colon cancer starts from a polyp, but not all polyps turn into colon cancer. The relationship between colon cancer and polyps is similar to the relationship between a caterpillar and a butterfly. We know that all butterflies come from caterpillars, but not all caterpillars turn into butterflies; a lot of them become moths! If we wanted to eliminate all the butterflies from this planet, the best plan would be to hunt down caterpillars. Well, same thing here. The purpose of screening is to go "polyp hunting." Along the way, other diseases of the lower intestine may be detected as well, such as ulcerative colitis (see number 7, page 10).

2. Screen by Age Forty-five

If you are reading this and you're under the age of thirty, then it's recommended that you begin screening for colorectal cancer (cancer of the colon and/or rectum) *at* age thirty, screening every two years thereafter. But chances are, you're well past thirty, and you're reading this book because you're thinking about preventing a cancer you feel is associated with aging. So don't panic. Beginning annual screening for colon cancer *by* age forty-five is still fine. Uh-oh—are you over forty-five? Well, get thee to your annual physical and request that screening begin now. It's certainly better than no screening at all.

Anyone aged forty-five or older is at risk for colorectal cancer (colon and/or rectal) cancer, although it occurs occasionally in people who are thirty-something. In the general population, one in twenty people without any known risk factors for colorectal cancer will develop it. Known risk factors for colorectal cancer include a history of ulcerative colitis, a family history of colorectal cancer, a history of benign tumors in the colon or rectum (called polyps), a diet high in fat and low in fiber, and *possibly* a family history of breast or ovarian cancers (this, however, is hotly debated).

3. Know the Alarm Signs

No matter how old you are, or how recently you've been screened for evidence of colon cancer, there are certain "red flag" symptoms that warrant an immediate investigation by a gastrointestinal specialist, called either a colorectal surgeon or a gastroenterologist. Alarming symptoms don't necessarily mean you have something serious; they mean you should *rule out* something serious. The word that distinguishes alarming symptoms from chronic symptoms is "sudden." If you're between forty-five and fifty-five, and you *suddenly* notice the onset of any of the following symptoms, don't wait and see what happens. Get yourself to a doctor's office as soon as possible, where you can be referred for testing or to a specialist.

Symptoms that may indicate a more serious illness, such as cancer, include:

- changes in bowel habits

- changes in stool consistency

- black stool or dark red blood in the stool (black stools indicate bleeding from the stomach; dark red blood in the stool means the bleeding is from the lower intestine)

- anemia (this could mean that you're bleeding from your gastrointestinal tract)

- persistent abdominal pain (nothing makes it go away)

- new and unusual symptoms (particularly if you're between ages forty-five and fifty or over sixty-five)

- weight loss (you've lost at least 5 to 10 pounds in the last month without trying)

The following symptoms indicate there is a problem in your upper gastrointestinal tract:

- vomiting (particularly vomiting blood)

- bloody saliva

- noticing that food or liquid is sticking in your throat (called dysphagia, or difficulty swallowing)

- feeling full after a few bites (if it's accompanied by heartburn, pain, bloating, and nausea)

4. Request the Appropriate Screening Tests

If you are between ages thirty and forty-five, request the following exams as part of your annual physical:

- *Visual examination of your rectal area.* Here, your doctor looks for visible signs of irritation or inflammation in that area.

- *Digital rectal exam.* Yes, you *will* survive this. Chevy Chase, in the first *Fletch* movie, does a nice demonstration of a patient having this exam. This is the one where a doctor puts on the ol' rubber gloves, lubricates a finger, and sticks the finger right up there to feel for unusual things: swelling, the state of your "sphincter muscles," and for tenderness, which could be a sign of anal fissures or inflammation. Although this was once the gold standard for checking prostate health in men, the PSA blood test (a blood test that detects early prostate cancer) and ultrasound are used to confirm the results of this exam for accuracy. In women, the cervix, a bit of the uterus, and a condition known as rectocele (when the rectum bulges slightly into the vagina) can be checked. Anyone engaging in regular anal sex should have this exam annually, too.

- *Anoscope exam.* Here, a short lighted tube, similar but much shorter than a sigmoidoscope (see page 7) is inserted to look for signs of inflammation or polyp growth. Since a sigmoidoscopy is much more accurate, however, many specialists recommend you skip this and go directly to sigmoidoscopy every two years until that magic forty-fifth birthday.

- *Occult blood test*. Also known as fecal occult blood test (FOBT), this test checks for "hidden" blood in the stools. (*Occult* means "hidden.") You collect your own stool samples from three bowel movements in a row. If blood is found in the stool samples, you'll be referred for a colonoscopy. Certain things in your diet, some medications, or the presence of hemorrhoids (and especially an inflamed anus, called anusitis) could give you false positive results. The cost of this test ranges from $5 to $10. It detects less than 10 percent of small polyps, 30 to 50 percent of large polyps, and 40 to 50 percent of early stage colorectal cancers. In other words, it may not detect the presence of polyps or cancer.

If you are over age forty-five, you should request all the above, plus:

- *Sigmoidoscopy*. Here, a short tube with a lighted microscope on the end is inserted about 6 inches into your rectum. The lining of your colon can be examined this way, and any inflammation or polyps (growths that can be benign or malignant) can be seen. Some doctors use a flexible sigmoidoscope, which is longer (about 2 feet), but since a colonoscope reveals more, there's not much point. This test costs about $100 and detects 30 to 45 percent of small polyps and 35 to 50 percent of large polyps or early stage cancers.

- *Colonoscopy*. (Alternate every year between this and the sigmoidoscopy!) Prior to this test, you'll need to be "cleaned out" with laxatives and a liquid diet so that the field of vision is clear. A long fiber-optic, lighted tube (approximately 5 feet or 165 cm long) is inserted into the colon usually while you are under sedation. This enables the doctor to view all sides of the colon, looking for polyps, inflammation, and so on, and allows growths to be removed during the procedure — a particular bonus. A more effective and newer colonoscope is a video colonoscope; this allows a clearer view (in color) on video. More polyps are found with this tool than with a fiber-optic colonoscope. This test costs between $500 to $1,000 in the United States and detects a whopping 85 percent of small polyps and about 97 percent of large polyps and early stage cancers. Because of the high cost of this test, however, it may not be accessible to everyone, depending on insurance coverage and income bracket. Many HMOs, for example, restrict colonoscopy to high-risk patients only, even though it is really a prevention tool. Clearly, access to colonoscopy should be made available for anyone who is at risk for colon cancer.

5. Request Colonoscopy in Place of Barium Enema

In light of far more accurate screening tools, such as sigmoidoscopy and colonoscopy, barium enemas are fast becoming the dinosaurs of colon cancer screening. You still need to be "cleaned out" via laxatives and a liquid diet the night before, but it may be harder to get your bowel movements back to normal after the test because the barium can dry out in the colon and become as hard as concrete. All in all, the black-and-white, two-dimensional images produced by barium x-ray are simply not as accurate as those seen in 3-D color via colonoscopy or sigmoidoscopy, and you are exposed to a small amount of radiation to boot. This test is also pretty costly, at $300 to $500. Since the test is expensive, and the results may be inconclusive, if not inaccurate—which would warrant colonoscopy anyway—most experts today recommend skipping the barium x-ray and going directly to colonoscopy.

6. Know the Rules for People with Inflammatory Bowel Disease

Inflammatory bowel disease (IBD) is a serious, chronic condition that can be life threatening in extreme cases. IBD means that one or more parts of your small or large intestine is inflamed, causing symptoms that range from unpleasant but manageable to severe and debilitating.

When inflammation and/or ulceration is confined to the inner lining of the colon (colitis) and rectum (proctitis), you have what's known as ulcerative colitis. This inflammation usually starts in the rectum and may spread throughout the colon. Because it's inflamed, the colon will not be able to do what it was designed to do: hold your solid waste. As a result, it will need to empty waste as soon as it receives it; you'll experience this as diarrhea. The inflammation will cause the cells that line the colon to slough off or die, which may cause open sores on the lining (ulcers), which could then form pus or mucus. So the diarrhea is often tinged with blood, pus, or mucus.

When the inflammation goes beyond the lining into the actual walls of the intestine, you have what's known as Crohn's disease, which usually attacks a part of the GI tract above the colon, in the ileum. For this reason, Crohn's disease is also known as ileitis or regional enteritis. But Crohn's disease can also attack the colon and/or other parts of the gastrointestinal tract.

If your intestines were a trench coat, ulcerative colitis would be confined to the lining of the coat below the belt, or ileum; that is, the lining of the colon and rectum. Crohn's disease would affect the *entire coat* starting at the belt, and possibly all the way up to the collar (the upper GI tract). Or it could start at the belt and affect everything below it (the lower GI tract). Think of the belt as the official separation between the upper and lower GI tract.

The risk of colon cancer is about thirty-two times higher if you have ulcerative colitis. That's because ulcerative colitis can cause the cells that line the colon to become precancerous (known as dysplasia). If only your rectum or the lower part of your colon is involved, then your risk is not any higher than in the general population. Nevertheless, if you've had ulcerative colitis for more than eight years, you should be screened *annually* for evidence of dysplasia through sigmoidoscopy or colonoscopy. Tissue biopsies can be obtained through colonoscopy. If dysplasia is found, you may be offered the option of a colectomy (surgical removal of the colon) to prevent the spread of precancerous cells and the development of full-blown colon cancer.

7. Know the Symptoms of Ulcerative Colitis

You may have ulcerative colitis, and be at increased risk of colon cancer—but never have been officially diagnosed with this illness. So be aware of these symptoms that may indicate this condition.

Abdominal cramps combined with bloody diarrhea (which could contain mucus and/or pus) and frequent, *urgent* bowel movements are the most common signs of ulcerative colitis. The diarrhea usually strikes immediately after meals or at night. Some people may also lose control of their bowel movements (called fecal incontinence) or pass stool in the belief that it is just gas. Obviously, these symptoms can interfere with many of your daily activities, including sleeping. Not all people suffer from severe symptoms; it really depends on where the inflammation is. Sometimes it's confined to the rectum, or one side of the colon rather than the entire colon.

Yet when symptoms *are* severe, you can suffer from all of the following:

- fatigue
- weight loss
- loss of appetite and/or nausea
- rectal bleeding
- malnutrition (mainly due to the loss of fluids and nutrients)
- anemia (from bleeding)

The same factors that trigger your immune system to attack your bowel tissue can also cause it to attack other body tissues, resulting in complications such as skin lesions, arthritis, inflammation of the eyes, or liver disorders, including jaundice and cirrhosis (which could necessitate a liver transplant).

In severe but rare cases, the colon enlarges and distends, known as toxic megacolon. This will cause fever, abdominal pain, dehydration, and malnutrition. In this case, surgery is necessary to prevent the colon from rupturing.

8. Know the Symptoms of Crohn's Disease

The symptoms of Crohn's disease are similar to ulcerative colitis: abdominal cramps (usually in your lower right side) and diarrhea, resulting in rectal bleeding, anemia, weight loss, and fever (rarely a symptom in ulcerative colitis unless the colon enlarges). The fever may make it easy for Crohn's disease to be confused with infectious diarrhea.

Because Crohn's disease attacks the intestinal walls and can occur higher up the gastrointestinal tract, obstruction can take place due to the narrowing of passageways (they swell and develop scar tissue). Fistulas ("ulcer tunnels" between tissues) can arise around the bladder, rectum, anus, or vagina. These tunnels can become infected and filled with pus. They are a common complication of Crohn's disease and often are associated with pockets of infection or abscesses (infected areas of pus).

As with ulcerative colitis, the autoimmune nature of Crohn's disease can also cause other body parts to become inflamed, including joints, skin, eyes, and mouth. Kidney stones and gallstones are also complications related to Crohn's.

Getting an Accurate Diagnosis of Ulcerative Colitis or Crohn's

Since the symptoms of both ulcerative colitis and Crohn's are virtually indistinguishable, the only way to tell which disease you have is for a specialist to obtain a tissue sample. This sample will then be analyzed under a microscope by a pathologist—preferably one who subspecializes in gastroenterology. A GI specialist can get a tissue sample through a procedure known as sigmoidoscopy (see page 7) or a colonoscopy.

Your doctor will also want to collect a stool sample to rule out infections or parasites, which can also cause mucus- or pus-tinged diarrhea. And finally, blood tests will confirm whether you're anemic or have a high white blood cell count (a sign of inflammation).

9. Understand What Genetic Testing for Colon Cancer Means

Yes, you can be tested for a "colon cancer gene," but the presence of a genetic mutation for colon cancer does not mean you will get colon cancer, nor does the *absence* of a genetic mutation mean that you will *not* get colon cancer. Therefore, genetic screening for colon cancer is not mean- ingful information for most people. And the stress a positive test can generate may cause more harm than good! If you do test positive for one of the types of colon cancer genes (or, more accurately, genetic mutations), you are encouraged to screen more frequently than people who do not have a genet- ic mutation for colon cancer.

Colon Cancer Genes

There is one type of colon cancer that does not originate from polyps, known as hereditary non-polyposis colorectal cancer (HNPCC). This is a hereditary colorectal cancer that strikes at about age forty-five. People with the gene for this cancer may also be more at risk for cancers of the uterus, bladder, ureter (the orifice out of which we urinate), pan- creas, and stomach. Roughly 5 percent of colorectal cancer is due to an HNPCC gene mutation.

A second gene mutation has been discovered in roughly 6 percent of the Ashkenazi Jewish population (Jews of

Eastern European descent). If you are not Jewish, it is exceedingly rare to test positive for this second kind of mutation.

Finally, less than 1 percent of colon cancer, known as familial adenomatous polyposis (FAP), which is characterized by hundreds of polyps, is linked to a rare genetic mutation.

10. Know the Downside of Genetic Testing for Colon Cancer

Some of the following questions regarding testing for the colon cancer gene should be considered:

1. *Who owns this information?* It is currently unclear whether people who test positive for a cancer gene mutation can keep the information confidential.

2. *How will this information be used?* The film *Gattaca* dramatizes the results of a genetically obsessed culture. In this film, one's genetic makeup determines one's eligibility for education, employment, and social status, even though the film's protagonist makes it clear that "genoism" (a word from the film, which meant discrimination against people with genetic "defects" or mutations) is against the law. *Gattaca* shows us a world that is not as futuristic as we might hope; a world where every strand of hair or eyelash serves as one's genetic résumé.

3. *Is getting tested harmful?* It can be, depending on how you're interpreting the news, or who is interpreting it for you. If you have inadequate genetic counseling (which happens a lot!), critics of genetic testing state that misunderstood genetic information can do enormous damage.

Consider these factors before you undergo genetic testing for colon cancer:

- *Testing negative.* Testing negative is never a "true negative," since the test is not an accurate prediction of
  one's future health. Some people mistakenly interpret
  a negative result to mean that they will never develop
  any form of colon cancer. If other people in your family are being tested at the same time, the family members who test negative may suffer from "survivor's
  guilt" if other family members test positive.

- *Testing positive.* On the flip side, testing positive is not
  necessarily a guarantee of colon cancer, although there
  is certainly a greater likelihood of it. The issue of harm
  should be examined, in the context of whether a still
  healthy, presymptomatic person should sacrifice his or
  her emotional health. People who test positive are more
  likely to suffer from anxiety, depression, and hope-
  lessness; strained relationships with family members;
  and even employment and insurance discrimination.

- *Inadequate counseling.* Genetic testing for any kind of
  mutation demands proper counseling before and after
  testing. Without proper counseling, critics of testing
  compare handing out test results to handing a loaded
  gun to a child. But that is not their worst fear. *There
  are not enough counselors to go around.* In the United
  States, for example, roughly twelve million people
  could benefit from genetic counseling, but there are
  only a thousand trained genetic counselors, only forty
  of whom actually work in clinical cancer centers.

Eating Fiber and
Staying Regular

11. Understand Fiber

Fiber is the part of a plant your body can't digest. It comes in the form of both soluble fiber (which dissolves in water) and insoluble fiber (which does not dissolve in water but, instead, absorbs water). Soluble and insoluble fiber do differ, but they are equally beneficial.

Soluble fiber somehow lowers the "bad" cholesterol, or low-density lipoprotein (LDL), in your body. Experts aren't entirely sure how soluble fiber works its magic, but one popular theory is that it gets mixed into the bile secreted by the liver and forms a type of gel that traps the building blocks of cholesterol, thus lowering your LDL levels. It's akin to a spider trapping smaller insects in its web.

Insoluble fiber doesn't affect your cholesterol levels at all, but it does regulate your bowel movements. How does it do this? As the insoluble fiber moves through your digestive tract, it absorbs water like a sponge and helps to form your waste quickly into a solid form, making the stools larger, softer, and easier to pass. Without insoluble fiber, your solid waste just gets pushed down to the colon or lower intestine as usual, where it is stored and dried out until you're ready to have a bowel movement. High-starch foods are associated with drier stools. This is exacerbated when you "ignore the urge," as the colon will dehydrate the waste even more until it becomes hard and difficult to pass, a condition known as constipation. Insoluble fiber helps to regulate your bowel movements by speeding things along. Insoluble fiber increases the "transit time" by improving colon motility and limiting the time dietary toxins "hang around" the intestinal wall. This is why it can dramatically decrease your risk of colon cancer.

12. Know Your Sources of Soluble versus Insoluble Fiber

Good sources of soluble fiber include oats or oat bran, legumes (dried beans, peas, and soybeans), some seeds, carrots, oranges, bananas, and other fruits. One of the most beneficial forms of soluble fiber is the soybean, particularly for people with very high cholesterol. In addition, the soybean is also a phytoestrogen (plant estrogen) that is believed to lower the risks of estrogen-related cancers (for example, breast cancer), as well as relieve estrogen-loss symptoms associated with menopause.

Good sources of insoluble fiber are wheat bran, whole grains, skins from various fruits and vegetables, seeds, leafy greens, and cruciferous vegetables (cauliflower, broccoli, and brussels sprouts). One problem for many people is understanding what is truly "whole grain." For example, there is an assumption that because bread is dark or brown, it's more nutritious; this isn't so. In fact, many brown breads are simply enriched white breads dyed with molasses. ("Enriched" means that some nutrients lost during processing have been replaced.) High-fiber pita breads and bagels are available, but you have to search for them. A good rule is to simply look for the phrase "whole wheat," which means that the wheat is, indeed, whole—and not simply white bread with coloring or flakes of wheat fiber to make it look more substantial than it is.

What's in a Grain?

Most of us turn to grains and cereals to boost fiber intake, which experts recommend should be at about 25 to 35 grams per day. Use the following chart to help gauge whether you're getting enough insoluble fiber. If you're a little under par, an easy way to boost your fiber intake is to simply add pure wheat bran to your foods (available in health food stores or supermarkets). Three tablespoons of wheat bran is equal to 4.4 grams of fiber. Sprinkle 1 to 2 tablespoons onto cereals, rice, pasta, or meat dishes. You can also sprinkle it into orange juice or low-fat yogurt. It has virtually no calories, but it's important to drink a glass of water with your wheat bran, as well a glass of water after you've finished your wheat bran–enriched meal. (See number 14, page 23, for more information.)

Cereals	Grams of Fiber
Fiber First (½ cup)	15.0
Fiber One (½ cup)	12.8
All Bran* (½ cup)	10.0
Oatmeal (½ cup)	5.0
Raisin Bran (¾ cup)	4.6
Bran Flakes (1 cup)	4.4
Shreddies (⅔ cup)	2.7
Cheerios (1 cup)	2.2
Cornflakes (1¼ cups)	0.8
Special K (1¼ cups)	0.4
Rice Krispies (1¼ cups)	0.3

*Some generic All Bran cereals have up to 15 grams of fiber.

Breads *(based on 1 slice)*	Grams of Fiber
Rye	2.0
Pumpernickel	2.0
Twelve-grain	1.7
100% whole wheat	1.3
Raisin	1.0
Cracked wheat	1.0
White	0

Keep in mind that some of the newer high-fiber breads on the market today have up to 7 grams of fiber per slice. This chart is based on what is typically found in regular grocery stores.

13. Know the Fiber Content of Your Fruits and Veggies

Another easy way of boosting fiber content is to know how much fiber your fruits and vegetables pack per serving, and choose those that provide the most. All fruits, beans (legumes), and vegetables listed here show the amount of insoluble fiber, which is not only good for colon health, but for your heart. Some of these numbers may surprise you!

Fruit	Grams of Fiber
Raspberries (¾ cup)	6.4
Strawberries (1 cup)	4.0
Blackberries (½ cup)	3.9
Orange (1)	3.0
Apple (1)	2.0
Pear (½ medium)	2.0
Grapefruit (½ medium)	1.1
Kiwi (1)	1.0

Beans	Grams of Fiber
Green beans (1 cup)	4.0
White beans (½ cup)	3.6
Kidney beans (½ cup)	3.3
Pinto beans (½ cup)	3.3
Lima beans (½ cup)	3.2

Vegetables	Grams of Fiber
Baked potato with skin (1 large)	4.0
Acorn squash (½ cup)	3.8
Peas (½ cup)	3.0
Corn, canned creamed (½ cup)	2.7
Brussels sprouts (½ cup)	2.3
Asparagus (¾ cup)	2.3
Corn kernels (½ cup)	2.1
Zucchini (½ cup)	1.4
Carrots, cooked (½ cup)	1.2
Broccoli (½ cup)	1.1

14. Drink Water with Fiber

How many people do you know who say, "But I *do* eat tons of fiber and I'm still constipated!" Probably quite a few. The reason they remain constipated in spite of their high-fiber diets is because they are not drinking *water* with fiber. Water means *water*. Milk, coffee, tea, soft drinks, or juice are not a substitute for water. Unless you drink water with your fiber, the fiber will not "bulk up" in your colon to create the nice, soft bowel movements you so desire. Think of fiber as a sponge. Obviously, a dry sponge won't work. You must soak it with water in order for it to be useful. Same thing here. Fiber without water is as useful as a dry sponge. *You must soak your fiber!* So here is the fiber/water recipe:

- Drink two glasses of water with your fiber. This means having a glass of water with whatever you're eating. Even if what you're eating does not contain much fiber, drinking water with your meal is a good habit to get into!

- Drink two glasses of water after you eat.

There are, of course, other reasons to drink lots of water throughout the day. Some studies show that dehydration can lead to mood swings and depression, for example. Numerous health and beauty experts advise women to drink eight to ten glasses of water per day for several reasons: water helps you to lose weight, have well-hydrated, beautiful skin, and urinate regularly, which is important for bladder function (women, in particular, can suffer from bladder infections and urinary incontinence). By drinking water with your fiber, you'll be able to get up to that "eight glasses of water per day" in no time.

15. Recognize a Normal Bowel

The colon essentially acts as a solid waste container, drying out the waste that doesn't get absorbed further up. The nervous system controls the muscular contractions of your colon, which slowly move your waste downward, toward your rectum. You experience these stronger muscular contractions as "the urge." And once you feel the urge, you sit down, relax, and allow the gentle contractions to overtake you. The anal sphincter will open to allow the passage of stool.

The frequency of bowel movements varies from person to person. Although many North American sources say it's "normal" to move your bowels anywhere from a few times per day to a few times per week, if you're not having one to three large, bulky, soft but firm bowel movements per day, you probably have a tendency to be constipated. A normal stool is solid or "formed" but not hard, and certainly should not contain mucus or blood. The stools should pass without cramps, pain, or strain. Normal stools can pass noisily, however, since natural gas (called flatus—swallowed air [nitrogen] that gets trapped in the lower intestine) often comes out with the stools (or independently).

16. Understand Constipation

Constipation means that you are not experiencing an urge to move your bowels, and when you do so the stools are hard and difficult to pass. Generally, if more than three days have gone by since your last bowel movement, the colon will continue to dry out the stools and the stools will harden.

Most constipation is "functional" in that there is no disease or organic difficulty at work; it's a lifestyle problem, connected to ignoring the urge to go (if you're surrounded by public toilets, for example) or not allowing enough time in the morning to *create* the urge to go by drinking or eating something. If you ignore the urge too often, you may stop feeling an urge altogether (see number 20: Retrain Your Bowels, page 31). Studies comparing the bowel habits of North Americans to Africans show that the incidence of colon cancer is higher in North Americans, who have less frequent bowel movements than do Africans. We can learn from these studies, and modify our lifestyles accordingly. The idea is to find a happy medium, because chronic diarrhea is also dangerous to your health. In fact, it's far more troublesome than chronic constipation.

If your constipation is a more sudden or recent occurrence in your life, then there could be other causes, such as:

- Hypothyroidism (low-functioning thyroid). Request a thyroid stimulating hormone (TSH) test to check for thyroid function, if you suspect this.

- Pregnancy or changes in the menstrual cycle. It's not unusual for women to experience constipation at these times.

- Hot weather. When you're perspiring, and losing body fluid, you could become constipated.

- Stress. This is often the cause. (See "commuter constipation" on page 30.)

- Travel (changes in schedule, diet, and time zones can interfere with regularity).

- Anal sores (this includes fissures, hemorrhoids, or herpes).

- Medications (particularly pain control medications in chronic illness).

- Periods of vomiting and diarrhea.

Chronic Constipation

Chronic constipation can have a variety of causes, including laxative abuse, diseases affecting body tissues, nerve or muscle control problems, inflammation, scarring or blockage in the lower intestine, spinal injuries, and prolonged bed rest or being bedridden (especially in seniors). Lack of exercise and poor diet, though, are the most common reasons for this condition.

Hemorrhoids

The straining caused by chronic constipation can lead to hemorrhoids, also known as "piles." These are swelling of tissue attached to, or arising from, certain locations of the anal canal and covered by the lining (mucosa) of the anal canal. A classic symptom of hemorrhoids is finding bright red blood squirting into the toilet water. Blood from hemorrhoids can also be seen covering your stool, in the toilet bowl, or on toilet paper. Sometimes an internal hemorrhoid is large enough that it protrudes through your rectum, and hangs outside the body. This is known as a protruding hemorrhoid. Since bleeding is a problem with internal hemorrhoids, you can become anemic.

To find some relief, try warm tub or sitz baths (when the water just covers your hips) several times a day. Don't use anything in the water except a little baking soda (optional), and don't stay in longer than about ten minutes. Stool softeners may help you pass stool more comfortably, while ice packs will help reduce swelling (ten minutes on/ten minutes off). Lying down with your hips elevated on a pillow may help. Over-the-counter medication such as Preparation H can also give you relief but won't shrink the hemorrhoid. If the problem does not resolve itself, and the hemorrhoid is painful, it is probably a blood clot, and the hemorrhoid can be removed in your doctor's office. Hemorrhoids are usually not painful, however.

17. Stay Regular Without Laxatives

If you're not moving your bowels at least once a day, you can probably change this by modifying your diet or lifestyle. Most often, *not* eating enough soluble fiber, *not* drinking enough water, and *not* getting enough exercise are the causes of constipation. Exercise helps to strengthen your abdominal muscles, and helps blood and oxygen circulate throughout your body, which simply makes *everything* work better. See the Exercise section for more details as well as Figure 2 for how to relieve constipation without drugs.

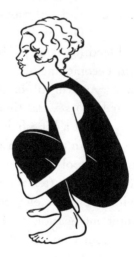

FIGURE 2

The Squat. By doing this exercise regularly, you can become more regular, too! You simply stand with your feet parallel to your hips and slowly squat down, making sure your weight is forward (rather than reeling backward or rolling your knees inward). You may need to practice a few times before you can do this comfortably. It's recommended that you "squat" twice a day to relieve constipation.

18. Know the Right Laxatives

The best way to know the "right" laxatives is to first know the *wrong* ones. You want to avoid anything that is a stimulant laxative. Stimulant laxatives work by stimulating the colon to contract, creating a bowel movement. You can easily become dependent on these substances, however, and you will soon be unable to move your bowels without such artificial means. Stimulant laxatives also include certain herbal laxatives, such as senna and cascara sagrada. Many herbalists maintain that cascara sagrada, unlike senna, is more of a tonic than a laxative and will not create a dependency; they believe, in fact, it may be helpful for your colon. Like other stimulant laxatives, though, it works by stimulating the colon to contract and create a bowel movement and, with too much use, dependency. As a result, many doctors strongly advise against cascara sagrada.

Meanwhile, there are several herbal teas and herbal concoctions that promote digestion and regularity through harmless spices or ingredients. You may have heard of acidophilus (liquid or powder); when used as a remedy for chronic constipation, it does not create dependency. In Ayurvedic medicine (an ancient Indian healing system), triphala is taken to promote regularity and good digestion. Triphala is a combination of three ancient Ayurvedic ingredients, haritaki, bibhitaki, and amalaki, and it can be found in most health food stores.

In addition, the following spices are good for digestion, and are not harmful to your colon in any way: licorice root, peppermint leaf, anise seed, yellow dock root, dandelion root, rose petals, coriander seed, celery seed, cinnamon bark, gingerroot, cardamom seed, clove bud, and black pepper.

If you must use an occasional laxative, the best kind are bulking agents (such as Metamucil, which is comprised of 90 percent insoluble fiber), which are sold as laxatives but are actually not laxatives per se. Adopting a "water with fiber routine" (see number 14, page 23,) will probably cure you of constipation without laxatives. Fifteen-gram fiber cereals with water are still the best remedy.

If nothing is working, and you haven't moved your bowels in five or six days, try inserting a glycerin suppository overnight and again in the morning. This should get things moving. If there's still no action, the next step is to try an enema, and after that, a mild laxative, such as milk of magnesia. If these don't work, you may have a bowel obstruction of some sort, so it would be wise to consult a good GI specialist.

19. Always Answer the Call of Nature

By simply obeying your urges, you can avoid constipation. Learning to suppress the urge to defecate can create what is called a "lazy bowel." When you feel the urge to defecate, drop what you're doing and get to the toilet. We all know ways of excusing ourselves to make or take "important calls." Why not make the call of nature the most important call of your day?

Another way to obey the call of nature is to give yourself enough time to receive the call in the first place. If you get out of bed in the morning and rush out the door immediately, you may be one of millions who suffers from "commuter constipation."

20. Retrain Your Bowels

For many, years of ignoring our natural urges and laxative dependency have made it impossible to "go it alone." Take heart: You can retrain your bowel to function correctly. Here's the recipe:

- Drink a glass of warm water in the morning as soon as you get up, and insert a glycerin suppository into your rectum.

- Move around a bit (make your bed, do some stretches, and so on) for about three or four minutes.

- Sit on the toilet and gently push for about two minutes. If nothing happens, get up and leave.

If you practice this routine every day for three to six months, you should be able to train your colon to have a bowel movement when you drink warm water in the morning. In other words, the warm water will stimulate your colon. Missing even a day of this routine could set you back weeks, though!

Eating Less Fat

21. Understand Fat

Fat is technically known as fatty acids, which are crucial nutrients for our cells. We cannot live without fatty acids, or fat. If you looked at each fat molecule carefully, you'd find it contains three different kinds of fatty acids:

- saturated (solid)
- monounsaturated (less solid, with the exception of olive and peanut oils)
- polyunsaturated (liquid)

When you see the term *unsaturated fat*, this refers to either monounsaturated or polyunsaturated fats.

These three fatty acids combine with glycerol to make what's chemically known as triglycerides. Each fat molecule is a link in a chain made up of glycerol, carbon atoms, and hydrogen atoms. The more hydrogen atoms that are on a specific chain, the more saturated or solid the fat.

The liver breaks down fat molecules by secreting bile (which is stored in the gallbladder). The liver also makes cholesterol. Too much saturated fat may cause your liver to overproduce cholesterol, while the triglycerides in your bloodstream will rise, perpetuating the problem.

Fat is a good thing—in moderation. But like all good things, most of us want too much of it. Excess dietary fat is by far the most damaging element in the Western diet. A gram of fat contains twice the calories as the same amount of protein or carbohydrate. Decreasing the fat in your diet and replacing it with more grain products, vegetables, and fruit is the best way to lower your risk of colon cancer and cardiovascular diseases. Fat in the diet comes from meats, dairy products, and vegetable oils. Other sources of fat include coconuts (60 percent fat), peanuts (78 percent fat), and avocados (82 percent fat). There are different kinds of fatty acids in these sources of fats: saturated, monounsaturated, and polyunsaturated. Finally, there is a fourth kind of fat in the diet: trans-fatty acids, which are a factory-made fat found in margarines.

Cutting through all this fat jargon, you can boil down fat into two categories: harmful fats and helpful fats (which the popular press often define as "good fats/bad fats").

Harmful Fats

The following are harmful fats because they can increase your risk of cardiovascular problems, as well as many cancers, including colon and breast cancers. These are fats that are fine in moderation, but harmful in excess (and harmless if not eaten at all):

- *Saturated fats.* These are solid at room temperature and stimulate cholesterol production in your body. In fact, the way that saturated fat looks prior to ingesting it is the way it will look when it lines your arteries. Foods high in saturated fat include: processed meat, fatty meat, lard, butter, margarine, solid vegetable shortening, chocolate, and tropical oils. (Coconut oil is more than 90 percent saturated.) Saturated fat should be consumed only in very low amounts.

- *Trans-fatty acids.* These are factory-made fats that behave just like saturated fat in your body. See number 22, page 38, for details.

Helpful Fats

These are fats that are beneficial to your health, and actually protect against certain health problems, such as cardiovascular disease. You are encouraged to use these fats more rather than less frequently in your diet. In fact, nutritionists suggest that you substitute these for harmful fats:

- *Unsaturated fat.* This is partially solid or liquid at room temperature. The more liquid the fat, the more unsaturated it is, which in fact *lowers* your cholesterol levels. This group of fats includes monounsaturated fats and polyunsaturated fats. Sources of unsaturated fats include vegetable oils (canola, safflower, sunflower, and corn), seeds, and nuts. Most plants produce unsaturated fats, with the exception of tropical plants, such as coconuts.

- *Fish fats (omega-3 oils).* The fats naturally present in fish that swim in cold waters (known as omega-3 fatty acids or fish oils) are all unsaturated. Again, unsaturated fats are good for you—they lower cholesterol levels, are crucial for brain tissue, and protect against heart disease. Look for cold-water fish such as mackerel, albacore tuna, salmon, and sardines.

22. Avoid Factory-Made Fats

An assortment of factory-made fats have been introduced into our diets, courtesy of food producers who are trying to give us the taste of fat without all the calories or harmful effects of saturated fats. Unfortunately, factory-made fats offer their own bag of horrors. That's because when a fat is made in a factory, it becomes a "trans-fatty acid," a harmful fat that *not only* raises the level of "bad" cholesterol (LDL, short for low-density lipoprotein) in your bloodstream, but lowers the amount of "good" cholesterol (HDL, short for high-density lipoprotein) that's already there.

How does a "trans-fatty acid" come into being? Trans-fatty acids are what you get when you make a liquid oil, such as corn oil, into a more solid or spreadable substance, such as margarine. Trans-fatty acids, you might say, are the "road to hell, paved with good intentions." Someone, way back when, thought that if you could take the "good fat"— unsaturated fat—and solidify it, so it could double as butter or lard, you could eat the same things without missing the spreadable fat. That sounds like a great idea. Unfortunately, to make an unsaturated liquid fat more solid, you have to add hydrogen to its molecules. This is known as hydrogenation, the process that converts liquid fat to semisolid fat. That ever-popular chocolate bar ingredient, "hydrogenated palm oil" is a classic example of a trans-fatty acid. Hydrogenation also prolongs the shelf life of a fat, which can oxidize when exposed to air, causing rancid odors or flavors. Deep-frying oils used in the restaurant trade are generally hydrogenated.

What's Wrong with Trans-fatty Acids?

Trans-fatty acids are sold as polyunsaturated or monounsaturated fats with a line of advertising copy such as: "Made from polyunsaturated vegetable oil." The problem is, in your body, they are treated as saturated fats. So trans-fatty acids are saturated fats in disguise. The advertiser may, in fact, say that the product contains "no saturated fat" or is "healthier" than the comparable animal or tropical oil product with saturated fat. So be careful out there—*read your labels*. The magic word you're looking for is "hydrogenated." If the product lists a variety of unsaturated fats (monounsaturated X oil, polyunsaturated Y oil, and so on), keep reading. If the word *hydrogenated* appears, count that product as a saturated fat; your body will!

Margarine versus Butter

There's an old tongue twister: "Betty Botter bought some butter that made the batter bitter; so Betty Botter bought more butter that made the batter better." Are we making our batters bitter or better with margarine? It depends.

Since the news of trans-fatty acids broke in the late 1980s, margarine manufacturers began to offer some less "bitter" margarines; some contain no hydrogenated oils, while others much smaller amounts. Margarines with less than 60 percent to 80 percent oil (9 to 11 grams of fat) will contain 1 to 3 grams of trans-fatty acids per serving, compared to butter, which is 53 percent saturated fat. You might say it's a choice between a bad fat and a *worse* fat.

It's also possible for a liquid vegetable oil to retain a high concentration of unsaturated fat when it's been partially hydrogenated. In this case, your body will metabolize this as some saturated fat and some unsaturated fat.

Fake Fat

We have artificial sweeteners; why not artificial fat? This question has led to the creation of an emerging yet highly suspicious ingredient: *fat substitutes*, designed to replace real fat and hence reduce the calories from real fat without compromising the taste. This is done by creating a fake fat that the body cannot absorb.

One of the first fat substitutes was Simplesse, an all-natural fat substitute, made from milk and egg-white protein, which was developed by the NutraSweet Company. Simplesse apparently adds 1 to 2 calories per gram instead of the usual 9 calories per gram from fat. Other fat substitutes simply take protein and carbohydrates and modify them in some way to simulate the textures of fat (creamy, smooth, and so on). All these fat substitutes help to create low-fat products.

A calorie-free fat substitute is being promoted called olestra, developed by Procter & Gamble. It's currently being test-marketed in the United States in a variety of savory snacks such as potato chips and crackers. Olestra is a potentially dangerous ingredient that most health experts feel can do more harm than good. Canada has not yet approved it.

Olestra is made from a combination of vegetable oils and sugar. Therefore, it tastes just like the real thing, but the biochemical structure is a molecule too big for your liver to break down. So, olestra just gets passed into the large intestine and is excreted. Olestra is more than an "empty" molecule, however. According to the FDA Commissioner of Food and Drugs, olestra may cause diarrhea and cramps and may deplete your body of vital nutrients, including vitamins A, D, E, and K, necessary for blood to clot. Indeed, all studies conducted by Procter & Gamble have shown this potential. If the FDA approves olestra for use as a cooking-oil substitute, you'll see it in every imaginable high-fat product. In a critique of the product published in the *University of California at Berkeley Wellness Letter* in 1996 (the year olestra was approved for test markets), another danger was cited. Instead of encouraging people to choose nutritious foods, such as fruits, grains, and vegetables, over high-fat foods, products like these encourage a high *fake*-fat diet that's still too low in fiber and other essential nutrients. And the no-fat icing on the cake is that these people could potentially wind up with a vitamin deficiency, to boot. Products such as olestra should make you nervous.

23. Cut Down on Carbohydrates and Glucose

A diet high in carbohydrates and sugar can also make you fat. That's because carbohydrates—meaning starchy stuff, such as rice, pasta, breads, or potatoes, and sugar—can be stored as fat when eaten in excess.

Carbohydrates can be simple or complex. Simple carbohydrates are found in any food that has natural sugar (honey, fruits, juices, vegetables, milk) and anything containing table sugar. Complex carbohydrates are more sophisticated foods that are made up of larger molecules, such as grain foods, starches, and foods high in fiber.

Normally, all carbohydrates when consumed convert into glucose (the technical term for "simplest sugar"). All your energy comes from glucose in your blood—also known as blood glucose or blood sugar: your body fuel. When your blood sugar is used up, you feel weak and tired—and hungry. But what happens when you eat more carbohydrates than your body can use? You store those extra carbohydrates as fat. What we also know is that the rate at which glucose is absorbed by your body from carbohydrates is affected by other parts of your meal, such as protein, fiber, and fat. If you're eating only carbohydrates and no protein or fat, for example, they will convert into glucose more quickly—to the point where you may feel mood swings, as your blood sugar rises and falls.

Nutritionists advise that daily you should consume roughly 50 to 55 percent carbohydrates, 15 to 20 percent protein, and less than 30 percent fat for a healthy diet.

24. Understand Sugar

Sugars are found naturally in many foods you eat. The simplest form of sugar is glucose, which is what blood sugar, also called blood glucose is: your basic body fuel. You can buy pure glucose at any drugstore in the form of dextrose tablets. Dextrose is just "edible glucose." For example, when you see people having "sugar water" fed to them intravenously, dextrose is the sugar in that water. When you see "dextrose" on a candy bar label, it means that the candy bar manufacturer used "edible glucose" in the recipe.

Glucose is the baseline ingredient of all naturally occurring sugars, which include:

- *Sucrose*: table or white sugar, naturally found in sugar cane and sugar beets
- *Fructose*: the natural sugar in fruits and vegetables
- *Lactose*: the natural sugar in all milk products
- *Maltose*: the natural sugar in grains (flours and cereals)

When you ingest a natural sugar of any kind, you're actually ingesting one part glucose, and one or two parts of *another* naturally occurring sugar. For example, sucrose is biochemically constructed from one part glucose and one part fructose. So, from glucose it came, and unto glucose it shall return—once it hits your digestive system. The same is true for all naturally occurring sugars, with the exception of lactose. As it happens, lactose breaks down into glucose and an "odd duck" simple sugar, galactose (which I used to think was something in our solar system until I became a health writer). Just think of lactose as the "Milky Way" and you'll probably remember.

Simple sugars can get pretty complicated when you discuss their molecular structures. For example, simple sugars can be classified as monosaccharides (single sugars) or disaccharides (double sugars). But unless you're writing a chemistry exam on sugars, you don't need to know this confusing stuff: You just need to know that all naturally occurring sugars wind up as glucose once you eat them; glucose is carried to your cells through the bloodstream, and is used as body fuel or energy.

How long does it take for one of the above sugars to return to glucose? It greatly depends on the amount of fiber in your food, how much protein you've eaten, and how much fat accompanies the sugar in your meal. As stated in number 23, if you have enough energy or fuel, once that sugar becomes glucose, it can be stored as fat. And that's how—and why—sugar can make you fat.

Factory-Added Sugars

What you have to watch out for is *added sugar*; these are sugars that manufacturers add to foods during processing or packaging. Foods containing fruit juice concentrates, invert sugar, regular corn syrup, honey or molasses, hydrolyzed lactose syrup, or high-fructose corn syrup (made out of fructose highly concentrated through the hydrolysis of starch) all have added sugars. Many people don't realize, however, that pure, *unsweetened* fruit juice is still a potent source of sugar, even when it contains no added sugar. Extra lactose (naturally occurring sugar in milk products), dextrose ("edible glucose"), and maltose (naturally occurring sugar in grains) are also contained in many of your foods. In other words, the products may have naturally occurring sugars anyway, and then *more* sugar is thrown in to enhance consistency, taste, and so on. The best way to know how much sugar is in a product is to look at the nutritional label for "carbohydrates."

25. Learn to Interpret Food Labels

Since 1993, food labels have been complying with strict guidelines set out by the Food and Drug Administration (FDA) and the U.S. Department of Agriculture's (USDA) Food Safety and Inspection Service (FSIS). All labels list "Nutrition Facts" on the side or back of the package. The "% Daily Values" column tells you how high or low that food is in various nutrients, such as fat, saturated fat, and cholesterol. A number of 5 or less is "low"—good news if the product shows <5 for fat, saturated fat, and cholesterol—bad news if the product is <5 for fiber. Serving sizes are also confusing. Foods that are similar are given the same *type* of serving size defined by the FDA. That means that five cereals all weighing X grams per cup will share the same serving sizes.

Calories (how much energy) and calories from fat (how

much fat) are also listed per serving of food. Total carbohydrate, dietary fiber, sugars, other carbohydrates (which means starches), total fat, saturated fat, cholesterol, sodium, potassium, and vitamins and minerals are given in Percent Daily Values, based on the 2,000-calorie diet recommended by the U.S. government. (In Canada, Recommended Nutrient Intake [RNI] is used for vitamins and minerals, while ingredients on labels are listed according to weight, with the "most" listed first.)

That's not where the confusion ends—*or even begins*! You have to wade through the label's various claims and understand what they mean. For example, anything that says "X free" (as in sugar free, saturated-fat free, cholesterol free, sodium free, calorie free, and so on) means that the product indeed has "no X" or that "X" is so tiny, it is dietarily insignificant. This is not the same thing as a label that says "95 percent fat free." In this case, the product contains relatively small amounts of fat, but still has fat. This claim is based on 100 grams of the product. For example, if a snack food contains 2.5 grams of fat per 50 grams, it can be said to be "95 percent fat free."

A label that screams "low in saturated fat" or "low in calories" is *not* fat free or calorie free. It means that you can eat a large amount of that food without exceeding the Daily Value for that food. In potato-chip country, that could mean you can eat twelve potato chips instead of six. So if you eat the whole bag of "low-fat" chips, you're still eating a lot of fat. Be sure to check serving sizes.

"Cholesterol free" or "low cholesterol" means that the product doesn't have any, or much, animal fat (hence, dietary cholesterol). This doesn't mean "low fat." Pure vegetable oil doesn't come from animals but is still pure fat!

"Less and More"

Next are the "comparison claims," such as "fewer," "reduced," "less," "more," or my favorite—"light" (or worse, "lite"!). These words appear on foods that have been nutritionally altered from a previous version or a competitor's version. For example, Brand X Potato Chips–Regular may have much more fat than Brand X Potato Chips–Lite "With Less Fat than Regular Brand X." That doesn't mean that Brand X Lite is fat free, or even low in fat. It just means it's B percent *lower* in fat than Brand X Regular.

On the flip side, Brand Y may have a trace amount of calcium, while Brand Y– "Now with More Calcium" may still have a small amount of calcium, but 10 percent more than Brand Y. (In other words, you may still need to eat a hundred bowls of Brand Y before you get the daily requirement for calcium!)

To be light or "lite," a product has to contain either one-third fewer calories or half the fat of the regular product; or, a low-calorie or low-fat food contains 50 percent less calories or fat. Something that is "light in sodium" means it has at least 50 percent less sodium than the regular product, such as canned soup.

"Sugar Free"

When a label says "sugar free," it contains less than 0.5 grams of sugar per serving, while a "reduced-sugar" food contains at least 25 percent less sugar per serving than the regular product. If the label also states that the product is not a reduced- or low-calorie food, or it is not for weight control, there's enough sugar in there to make you think twice.

But sugar free in the language of labels simply means "sucrose free." That doesn't mean the product is *carbohydrate free*, as in: dextrose free, lactose free, glucose free, or fructose free. Check the labels for all things ending in "ose" to find out the sugar content; you're not just looking for sucrose. Watch out for "no added sugar," "without added sugar," or "no sugar added." This simply means: "We didn't put the sugar in, God did."

Finally, when you see the following claims, know what they mean before you purchase the food items:

- *Low calorie* actually means 40 calories or less per serving.

- *Low fat* actually means 3 grams of fat or less per serving.

- *Low cholesterol* actually means 20 mg of cholesterol or less per serving (in addition to saturated fat and total fat restrictions that may be in your diet).

26. Become More or Semivegetarian

It's estimated that at least 7 to 10 percent of North Americans practice some type of vegetarianism. Semi-vegetarians eat poultry, fish, eggs, and dairy foods. Pesco-vegetarians eat fish, eggs, and dairy foods; lacto-ovo-vegetarians eat eggs and dairy foods. Stricter forms of vegetarianism include ovo-vegetarians, who do not eat dairy but will consume eggs; lacto-vegetarians, who will not eat eggs but will eat dairy; and vegans, who will not eat any sort of animal-derived foods.

When you compare the health of vegetarians to that of the general population, vegetarians have lower rates of heart disease, colon cancer, colitis (inflammation of the colon), hypertension, Type 2 diabetes, and obesity. A 1997 report from the American Institute for Cancer Research's Diet and Cancer Project, *Food Nutrition and the Prevention of Cancer: A Global Perspective,* advises that a plant-rich, vegetarian-based diet is a significant factor in reducing the risk of colon cancer.

Keep in mind that becoming more vegetarian isn't a license to overdo it on high-fat, meatless foods. You should still choose lower-fat dairy products if you eat dairy. Some suggestions:

- Go for one or two fruits at breakfast, one fruit and two vegetables at lunch and dinner, and a fruit or vegetable snack between meals.

- Consume many differently colored fruits and vegetables. For color variety, select at least three differently colored fruits and vegetables daily.

- Put fruit and sliced veggies in an easy-to-use, easy-to-reach place (sliced vegetables in the fridge; fruit out on the table).

- Keep frozen and canned fruits and vegetables on hand to add to soups, salads, or rice dishes.

27. Adopt Some of These Fat-Cutting Tips

Cutting fat from your diet is, of course, easier said than done. I've collected the following fat-cutting tips from my network of nutritionists, who insist that adopting or remembering just a few of these tips can really help.

- Whenever you refrigerate foods containing animal fat (soups, stews, or curry dishes), skim the fat from the top before reheating and re-serving. A gravy skimmer also helps remove fats; the spout pours from the bottom, which helps the oils and fats to coagulate on top.

- Substitute something else for butter: yogurt (great on potatoes) or low-fat cottage cheese, or, at dinner, just dip your bread into olive oil with some garlic, Italian style. For sandwiches, any condiment without butter, margarine, or mayonnaise is fine. This includes mustard, yogurt, salsa, and so on.

- Powdered nonfat milk is in vogue again; it's high in calcium, low in fat. Substitute it for any recipe calling for milk or cream.

- Dig out fruit recipes for dessert. Treats such as sorbet with low-fat yogurt topping can be elegant.

- Season low-fat foods well. That way, you won't miss the flavor fat adds.

- Lower-fat protein comes from vegetable sources (whole grains and bean products); higher-fat protein comes from animal sources.

If you're preparing meat:

- Broil, grill, or boil meat instead of frying, baking, or roasting it. (If you drain fat and cook in water, baking/roasting is fine.)

- Trim off all visible fat from meat before and after cooking.

- Adding flour, bread crumbs, or other coatings to lean meat adds fat.

- Try substituting low-fat turkey meat for red meat.

28. Learn to Read Labels on Dairy Products

In North America, we consume a lot of milk, which is often a leading source of saturated fat in our diets. Know what you're getting:

- Whole milk is made up of 48 percent calories from fat.
- 2% milk gets 37 percent of its calories from fat.
- 1% milk gets 26 percent of its calories from fat.
- Skim milk is completely fat free.
- Cheese gets 50 percent of its calories from fat, unless it's skim milk cheese.
- Butter gets 95 percent of its calories from fat.
- Yogurt gets 15 percent of its calories from fat, unless it's nonfat.

29. Learn How to Substitute

By making the following substitutions, you can significantly lower your dietary fat:

Substitute	For
Veggie burgers or chicken breast sandwiches	Hamburgers
Ground turkey or tofu (soybean)	Ground beef
Yogurt, hummus, or reduced-fat margarine	Butter
Skim milk or 1% milk	Homogenized milk
Club soda or water	Soft drinks

30. Avoid Defeating All Your Best Nutritional Efforts

The American Institute for Cancer Research's Diet and Cancer Project, Food Nutrition and the Prevention of Cancer recommends that by avoiding the following, you'll decrease your risk of colon cancer:

- Avoid salted foods and table salt whenever possible; season your foods with herbs.

- Avoid eating food that was "left out" for long periods of time; the food can become contaminated with bacteria.

- Avoid eating perishable foods that were not refrigerated.

- Avoid unlabeled foods when traveling in undeveloped (or developing) countries, as contaminants, additives, and other residues are not properly regulated in these areas.

- Avoid charred food or meat and fish cooked over an open flame.

- Avoid cured or smoked meats.

- Avoid chewing tobacco or smoking.

Exercising

31. Understand What Exercise *Really* Means

Both the American and Canadian Cancer Societies state that people who are inactive have higher rates of colon cancer. The *1999 Report of the Ontario Expert Panel on Colorectal Cancer Screening*, the most recently published task force report in North America on strategies to prevent colon cancer, also cites physical inactivity as a chief risk factor for colon cancer.

The *Oxford Dictionary* defines exercise as "the exertion of muscles, limbs, etc., especially for health's sake; bodily, mental, or spiritual training." In the Western world, we have placed an emphasis on "bodily training" when we talk about exercise, completely ignoring mental and spiritual training. Only recently have Western studies begun to focus on the mental benefits of exercise. (It's been shown, for example, that exercise creates endorphins, hormones that make us feel good.) But we in the West do not encourage meditation or other calming forms of mental and spiritual exercise, which have also been shown to improve well-being and health.

Nor should we ignore all the many cultural traditions known to improve mental health and well-being, such as traditional dances, active prayers that incorporate physical activity, circles that involve community and communication, and even sweat lodges, believed to help rid the body of toxins through sweating. These are all forms of wellness activities that you should investigate.

32. Understand What "Aerobic" Means

If you look up the word *aerobic* in the dictionary, what you'll find is the chemistry definition: "living in free oxygen." This is certainly correct; we are all aerobes—beings that require oxygen to live. (Only a few life-forms, such as some bacteria, are anaerobic, meaning they can exist in an environment that has no oxygen.) All that jumping around and fast movement in aerobics class is done to create faster breathing, so we can take more oxygen into our bodies.

Why should we do this? Because the blood contains *oxygen!* The faster your blood flows, the more oxygen can flow to your organs. When your health care practitioner tells you to "exercise" or to take up "aerobic exercise," she's not referring solely to "increasing oxygen" but to exercising the heart muscle. The faster it beats, the better a "workout" it gets. If you already have heart disease, or are on medications that affect your heart, check with your doctor to make sure you are not overworking this vital organ.

Exercise is considered aerobic if it makes your heart beat faster than it normally does. When your heart is beating fast, you'll be breathing hard and sweating and ideally will officially be in your "target zone" or "ideal range."

There are specific calculations you can do to find this target range. One technique is to subtract your age from 220, then multiply that number by 60 percent. This will give you your "threshold level"—which means your heart should be beating X beats per minute for 20 to 30 minutes. If you multiply the number by 75 percent, you will find your "ceiling level"—which means your heart should not be beating faster than X beats per minute for 20 to 30 minutes. This is only an example, however. If you are on heart medications (for example, drugs that slow down your heart, known as beta-blockers), you'll want to make sure you discuss with your health professional what "target" to aim for.

Why You Want More Oxygen

When more oxygen is in your body, you burn fat, your breathing is enhanced, your blood pressure improves, and your heart works better—which benefits your entire body. One major advantage is regularity. Oxygen also lowers triglycerides and cholesterol, increasing high-density lipoproteins (HDLs), or the "good" cholesterol, while decreasing our low-density lipoproteins (LDLs), or the "bad" cholesterol. This means that your arteries will unclog and you may significantly decrease your risk of heart disease and stroke. More oxygen makes your brain work better, so you feel better. Studies show that depression is decreased when you increase oxygen flow into your body. Ancient techniques such as yoga, which specifically improve mental and spiritual well-being, achieve this by combining deep breathing and stretching, which improves oxygen and blood flow to specific parts of the body.

Exercise has been shown to dramatically decrease the incidence of many other diseases, including cancer. Some research suggests that cancer cells tend to thrive in an oxygen-depleted environment. The more oxygen in the bloodstream, the less hospitable you make your body to cancer. In addition, since many cancers are related to fat-soluble toxins, the less fat on your body, the less fat-soluble toxins your body can accumulate.

Burning Fat

The only kind of exercise that will burn fat is aerobic exercise because *oxygen burns fat*. If you were to go to your fridge and pull out some animal fat (chicken skin, red-meat fat, or butter), throw it in the sink, and light it with a match, it would burn. What makes the flame yellow is oxygen; what fuels the fire is the fat. That same process goes on in your body. The oxygen will burn your fat, and you increase the oxygen flow in your body by jumping around/increasing your heart rate, or employing an established deep-breathing technique.

33. Use the Borg's Rate of Perceived Exertion (RPE)

This is a way of measuring exercise intensity without finding your pulse, and because of its simplicity, it is now the recommended method for judging exertion. This Borg "scale," as it's dubbed, goes from 6 to 20. An extremely light activity may rate a "7," for example, while a very, very hard activity may rate a "19." Exercise practitioners recommend that you do a "talk test" to rate your exertion level. If you can't talk without gasping for air, you may be working too hard. You should be able to carry on a normal conversation throughout your activity. What's crucial to remember about RPE is that it is extremely subjective; one person's "7" may be another person's "10."

34. Find Other Ways to Increase Oxygen Flow

You can increase the flow of oxygen into your bloodstream without exercising your heart muscle by learning how to breathe deeply through your diaphragm. There are many yogalike programs and videos that can teach you this technique, which does not require you to jump around. The benefit is that you increase the oxygen flow into your bloodstream. This is better than doing nothing at all to improve your health, and has many physical benefits, according to a myriad of wellness practitioners. Deep breathing exercises can also help to strengthen digestion and keep you regular.

35. Start Active Living Instead of "Aerobic" Living

The term *aerobic activity* means that the *activity* causes your heart to pump harder and faster, and causes you to breathe faster, which increases oxygen flow. Endeavors such as cross-country skiing, walking, hiking, and biking are all aerobic. Exercise professionals hate the terms *aerobic activity* and *aerobics program* because they are not about what people do in their daily lives. Health promoters are replacing these terms with the phrase *active living*—because that's what becoming nonsedentary is all about. There are many ways you can adopt an active lifestyle. Here are some suggestions:

- If you drive everywhere, pick the parking space furthest away from your destination so you can work some daily walking into your life.
- If you take public transit everywhere, get off one or two stops early so you can walk the rest of the way to your destination.
- Choose stairs over escalators or elevators.
- Park at one side of the mall and then walk to the other side.
- Take a stroll after dinner around your neighborhood.
- Volunteer to walk the dog.
- On weekends, go to the zoo or get out to flea markets, garage sales, and so on.

36. Begin Weight-Bearing Activities

You're not exercising just to prevent colon cancer but to make your entire body stronger and more efficient. The side benefit of this is that you can prevent a whole host of health problems and cancers, including colon cancer. Weight-bearing activities are encouraged because they build bone mass and use up calories. For many people, this is a very desirable form of exercise because it makes you stronger, which has a powerful effect on your self-esteem and body image.

By increasing muscular strength, we increase flexibility and endurance. For example, you'll find that the first time you ride your bike from home to downtown, your legs may feel sore. Do that same ride ten times, and your legs will no longer be sore. That's what is meant by building endurance. Of course, you won't be as out of breath, either, which is another type of endurance.

Hand weights or resistance exercises (using rubber-band gadgets or pushing certain body parts together) help increase what's called lean body mass—body tissue that is not fat. That is why many people find their weight does not drop when they begin to exercise. As your muscles become bigger, however, your body fat decreases.

37. Avoid Hazardous Exercises

Some activities, such as wrestling or weight lifting, are usually brief in duration but very intense. As a result, people with certain health problems may not be able to participate. For example, if you have heart problems, diabetes, or are taking medications that can affect your heart, intense exercise is not recommended.

38. Start Slow

Reports show that one out of three American adults is overweight, a sign of growing inactivity. Some people are so put off by the health club scene that they become even more sedentary. This is similar to diet failure, where you become so demoralized that you "cheated" that you binge even more.

What's the definition of sedentary? *Not moving!* If you have a desk job or spend most of your time at a computer, in your car, or watching television (even if it *is* PBS or CNN), you are a sedentary person. If you do roughly twenty minutes of exercise less than once a week, you're relatively sedentary, and you need to incorporate some sort of movement into your daily schedule in order to be considered active. That movement can be anything: aerobic exercise, brisk walks around the block, or walking your dog. If you've been sedentary most of your life, there's nothing wrong with starting off with simple, even leisurely activities such as gardening, feeding the birds in a park, or a few simple stretches. Any step you make toward being more active is a crucial and important one. A 1998 *New England Journal of Medicine* article reported that low-intensity exercise such as walking was associated with lower rates of cancers, such as colon cancer and prostate cancer.

Experts also recommend that you find a friend, neighbor, or relative to get physical with you. When your exercise plans include someone else, you'll be less apt to cancel plans or make excuses for not getting out there.

39. Prepare for "Moving Day"

Choose an activity that's right for you. Whether it's walking, chopping wood, jumping rope, or folk dancing—pick something you enjoy. Just try not to let two days pass without doing some movement. You don't have to do the same thing each time, either. Vary your routine to avoid monotony. Just make sure that whatever activity you choose is continuous for the duration. Walking for two minutes, then stopping for three, isn't continuous. If you're elderly or ill, even a few minutes is a good start. If you're sedentary but otherwise healthy, aim for twenty to thirty minutes. Finally, it's also important to choose an activity that doesn't aggravate a preexisting health problem.

More Intense Activities	Less Intense Activities
Skiing	Stretching
Running	Golf
Jogging	Bowling
Stair-stepping or stair-climbing	Badminton
Trampolining	Strolling
Jumping rope	Cricket
Fitness walking	Sailing
Race walking	Swimming
Aerobics classes	
Roller-skating	
Ice-skating	
Biking	
Weight-bearing exercise	
Tennis	
Swimming	

40. Stretch

Ever watch a cat in action? Cats will never do anything before stretching. If stretching *is* your exercise, that's just fine; but even for other activities, do some stretching before and after in order to reduce muscle tightness. Here are four easy stretches anyone can incorporate into his or her day:

- *Shoulder rotations*: While breathing deeply and slowly, use a circular pattern to move the right shoulder, and then switch to the left. One minute per shoulder is a good start.

- *Upper back stretch*: While sitting or standing, you simply stretch your arms upward and slightly behind you, taking deep, slow breaths. With arms up, face your palms toward heaven and rotate your thumbs.

- *Arm circles*: While sitting or standing, extend your arms so you look like a cross, and then move your arms in circles, starting small and getting larger.

- *Abdominal stretches* are particularly useful for strengthening the colon.

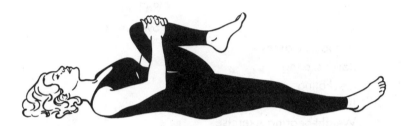

FIGURE 3

Knee-to-Chest—One Leg. As shown in Figure 3, this strengthens your abdominal muscles and, when combined with the Squat (see Figure 2, page 28), can effectively relieve chronic constipation. Lie on your back on the floor. Bend one knee and bring it in to the chest. Then just hug the leg, and slowly bring it toward your abdomen. Hold for a count of 10. Relax and repeat with alternate leg.

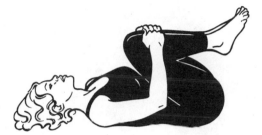

FIGURE 4

Knee-to-Chest—Both Legs. As shown in Figure 4, this is the same as the One-Leg version, only you bring both legs to the chest and hug them with both arms, bringing them gently toward your abdomen. Hold them there for the count of 10. Then relax and repeat.

Boosting Your Immune System

41. Know Phytochemicals and Functional Foods

Nutritional scientists have been slowly uncovering hidden treasures in our vegetables that are believed to help fight diseases. These are called phytochemicals, or "plant chemicals" (*phyto* is Greek for "plant").

In general, all green vegetables (such as broccoli, green beans, spinach, and lettuce) are for cellular repair. All red, orange, yellow, and even purple vegetables contain antioxidants thought to be the cancer-fighting "foot soldiers."

Functional foods refer to foods that have significant levels of biologically active disease-preventing or health-promoting properties. Dozens of phytochemicals have been identified and they range from isoflavones (found in soybeans) to saponins (found in spinach, potatoes, tomatoes, and oats).

Studies also show that cruciferous vegetables, such as cabbage, brussels sprouts, cauliflower, and broccoli, contain phytochemicals that especially protect against colon cancer. By simply eating a variety of fruits, grains, and vegetables, however, you will ensure your overall health.

42. Learn What Vitamins Are Good for Your Gut

It's believed that fruits and vegetables high in antioxidants, phytoestrogens (plant estrogens, found in soy), and lignins (a type of fiber) may also protect against a variety of cancers. Vitamin A and beta-carotene are associated with preventing or even reversing lung, larynx, colon, prostate, bladder, stomach, esophageal, and possibly breast cancer. Vitamins C, E, and selenium are associated with low rates of stomach and esophageal cancers, in particular. It's believed that vitamins C and E block the formation of carcinogenic compounds in the stomach, including polyps (see number 1, page 3). Vitamin D, which the body makes on its own when exposed to natural light, and calcium have been shown in some studies to protect against colorectal and breast cancers. Calcium apparently helps to absorb fecal bile acids, which experts believe promote tumors in the digestive tract. In fact, epidemiological studies show a higher incidence of colon and breast cancers in regions with less sunlight (although this could simply mean that where there's less sunlight, there's more sedentary living). And finally, epidemiological studies suggest folic acid may also lower the risk of colon cancer.

43. Know Sources of Vitamins and Minerals

It's easier to add a variety of vitamins and minerals to your diet if you know where to get them. Use this list to help you expand your nutrient intake:

- *Vitamin A/Beta-carotene*: Found in liver, egg yolks, whole milk, butter; beta-carotene—leafy greens, yellow and orange vegetables and fruits.

- *Vitamin B_6*: Found in meats, poultry, fish, nuts, liver, bananas, egg yolk, whole grains, legumes.

- *Vitamin B_{12}*: Found in meats, dairy products, eggs, liver, fish.

- *Vitamin C*: Found in citrus fruits, broccoli, green pepper, strawberries, cabbage, tomato, cantaloupe, potatoes, leafy greens.

- *Vitamin D*: Found in fortified milk, butter, leafy green vegetables, egg yolk, fish oils, butter, liver; also skin exposure to sunlight.

- *Vitamin E*: Found in nuts, seeds, whole grains, vegetable and fish-liver oils.

- *Vitamin K*: Found in leafy greens, corn and soybean oils, liver, cereals, dairy products, meats, fruits.

- *Calcium*: Found in milk and dairy products, leafy greens, broccoli, clams, oysters, almonds, walnuts, sunflower seeds, legumes, tofu; softened bones of canned fish (sardines, mackerel, salmon).

- *Copper*: Found in liver, shellfish, nuts, legumes, water.

- *Folic acid*: Found in liver (limit to 1 serving per week), eggs, leafy green vegetables, yeast, legumes, whole grains, nuts, fruits (bananas, orange juice, grapefruit juice), vegetables (broccoli, spinach, asparagus, brussels sprouts).

- *Iron*: (Heme iron is easily absorbed by the body; nonheme iron not as easily absorbed, so should be taken with vitamin C.) Heme iron is found in liver, meat, and poultry; nonheme iron is found in dried fruit, seeds, almonds, cashews, enriched and whole grains, legumes, and green leafy vegetables.

- *Niacin*: Found in grains, meats, nuts.

- *Zinc*: Found in oysters, seafood, meat, liver, eggs, whole grains, wheat germ.

44. Understand the Impact of Stress on Your Immune System

Since your immune system can be affected by stress, it's important to understand what is meant by "stress." Generally, it's defined as a negative emotional experience associated with biological changes that allow you to adapt to it. For example, in response to stress, your adrenal glands pump out "stress hormones" that speed up your body functions: Your heart rate increases and your blood sugar levels rise so that glucose can be diverted to your muscles in case you have to run. This is known as the "fight-or-flight" response.

The problem with stress hormones in the twenty-first century is that the fight-or-flight response usually isn't necessary, since most stress is emotional. Occasionally, a person may need to flee from a bank robber or mugger, but most of us just want to flee from our jobs or our kids! In other words, our stress hormones actually put a physical strain on our bodies, and can lower our resistance to disease. Initially, stress hormones stimulate the immune system; but after the stressful event has passed, they can suppress immune function.

Stress can affect every part of your body from head to toe, causing:

- headaches

- gastrointestinal problems

- bladder problems
- cardiovascular problems
- back pain
- high blood pressure
- high cholesterol

In general, you feel stress when you experience negative events; uncontrollable or unpredictable events; or ambiguous events (versus clear-cut situations). But how stressed you become has much to do with your personality as well. For example, if you have a negative outlook on life, you'll probably feel more stress than someone with a positive outlook.

Strategies for coping also vary. Some people like to avoid stress and minimize the problem. This has short-term benefits; but, over the long term, stress does not disappear. People who confront stress in the short term will feel more anxious at first, but will probably feel relief in the long term when factors causing stress are addressed. People who suffer less stress-related health problems frequently use humor, spiritual support, and social networking to deal with tension.

45. Reduce Lifestyle Stress

By reducing everyday lifestyle stresses, you're giving your immune system a boost. Stress reduction depends entirely on the source of your stress. The only way to control stress that is *beyond* your control is to shift your response to stress. For many of us, this takes time, and it may require some work with a qualified counselor.

If you are the source of your own stress, because you're too hard on yourself, or are a perfectionist, you need to work on lowering your self-expectations and forgiving yourself for not being faultless. Again, working with a therapist or counselor may help. In the meantime, here are some suggestions for reducing some sources of daily stress:

- *Isolate the exact source of stress* and see if there's a solution. (Taking the time to think about what, in fact, the real problem is can work wonders.)

- *See the humor in difficult situations,* and try to look at lessons learned instead of beating yourself up.

- *When times get tough, surround yourself with supportive people*: close friends, family members, and so on.

- *Don't take things so personally.* When people don't respond to you the way you'd like, consider other factors. For instance, maybe the other person has problems unrelated to you that are affecting her behavior.

- *Focus on something pleasant in the future,* such as a vacation, and allow yourself time to daydream, plan, and so on.

- *Just say "no."* If you can't take on that "small favor" or extra task, just politely say, "I'd love to, but it's impossible. . . ."

- *Take time out for yourself.* Spend some time alone and block everyone out once a week or so. This is a great time to just go for a long walk and get in a little exercise.

- *Lists.* Some people find list-making really helps; others find it is just another chore in and of itself. But if you haven't been a list-maker, try it. It might help you get a little more focused and organized on the tasks at hand.

- *Look into some alternative healing systems,* such as massage, or Chinese exercises, such as qi gong (pronounced "chi kong") or tai chi.

46. Reduce Occupational Stress

There are a number of sources of occupational stress, which include stress from superiors or coworkers (these are often personality clashes); commuter stress and long hours; and real occupational hazards that affect your health or quality of life.

If you're working with people with whom you cannot get along, or with people who cause you stress, consider changing jobs or even changing positions within the same company; this may be one way to eliminate a major source of stress. Commuting frustration and long hours can be addressed by looking at ways to telecommute or job-share.

One of the most important ways to reduce occupational stress is to lessen your exposure to occupational hazards. Workplaces using chemicals that are classified as hazardous by the appropriate government bodies must publicize this information to all employees, detailing the relevant components, hazards, and handling instructions specific to each chemical.

Working in a human-friendly environment can reduce numerous occupational stresses. Try to get some of these policies implemented at your workplace:

1. *Flexible working hours.* This can mean a variety of options that include banking time during off-peak hours; tailoring a shift or schedule that works better for you; part-time schedules; job-sharing; and longer breaks when necessary.

2. *Telecommuting.* Working from home at least some of the time can help to reduce stress by eliminating commutes. Obviously, certain jobs are more conducive to this than others. But if you use a computer and telephone, and have meetings with people, there's no reason why you can't work from home.

3. *Affordable infant and child care at or near the workplace.* Often these day-care facilities are offered at a reduced or no cost to employees. (Some companies even provide transportation to and from the day-care facility, but this is a rare situation.)

4. *Adequate breaks during the workday.* Frequent, short breaks contribute to stress reduction and greater productivity.

5. *Comfortable, private facilities on-site.* These are private rooms or quarters employees can go to for resting due to illness; meditation or stress relief; or even stretching during the workday. These facilities need not be fancy, and can take the form of a rest room (what old-fashioned washrooms *used* to have) consisting of a private room within a men's or ladies' washroom that has a small cot or comfortable couch, first-aid kits, and so on, for employees to use during the workday. Both men and women should have equal access to such facilities.

6. *Zero tolerance for sexism, prejudice against lifestyle preference, and racism.* That means no jokes about gender or gender preference, race, or ability.

7. *A clean workplace.* All employees have the right to clean washrooms, smoke-free environments, and hazard-free surroundings (for example, no asbestos).

8. *Publicized information regarding employee rights and policies.* All workers should understand their rights regarding leave policies, hazards, and so on.

47. Stay Tuned in to "Immune Boosters"

Five years ago, few people had even heard of immune boosters. Today, many substances, such as echinacea and zinc, are as popular as vitamin C. Here's an overview of some of the well-known immune boosters, substances that stimulate your immune system or strengthen it to help fight disease.

- *Echinacea.* This is a flower that belongs to the sunflower family. Echinacea is believed to increase the number of cells in your immune system to fight off disease.

- *Essiac.* This is a mixture of four herbs comprising Indian rhubarb, sheepshead sorrel, slippery elm, and burdock root. Essiac is believed to strengthen the immune system, improve appetite, supply essential nutrients to the body, possibly relieve pain, and ultimately, prolong life.

- *Ginseng.* This is a root used in Chinese medicine, but it's believed to enhance your immune system and boost the activity of white blood cells.

- *Green tea.* This is a popular Asian tea made from a plant called *Camellia sinensis.* The active chemical in green tea is epigallocatechin gallate (EGCG). It is believed that green tea neutralizes free radicals, which are carcinogenic. It is considered to be an anticancer tea—particularly for stomach, lung, and skin cancers.

- *Iscador* (mistletoe). Iscador is made through a fermentation process, using different kinds of mistletoe, a plant known for its white berries. Popular as an antitumor treatment in Europe, it's believed that Iscador works by enhancing the immune system and inhibiting tumor growth.

- *Pau d'arco* (Taheebo). This usually comes in the form of a tea made from the inner bark of a tree called Tabebuia. It's believed to be a cleansing agent; it can be used as an antimicrobial agent, and is said to stop tumor growth.

- *Wheatgrass*. This is grass grown from wheat-berry seeds, and it is rich in chlorophyll. Its juice contains over a hundred vitamins, minerals, and nutrients, and is believed to contain a number of cancer-fighting agents and have immune-boosting properties.

According to *A Guide to Unconventional Cancer Therapies*, a renowned booklet used by North American cancer patients seeking alternative treatment for cancer (published by the Ontario Breast Cancer Information Exchange Project, a Canadian government initiative), the following spices are said to be anticancer agents.

- garlic
- turmeric
- onions
- black pepper
- asafetida
- pippali
- cumin and poppy seeds

- kandathiipile
- neem flowers
- mananthakkali, drumstick, and basil leaves
- ponnakanni
- parsley

48. An Aspirin a Day
May Keep Colon Cancer Away

There is some research to support that taking one aspirin daily may reduce the number of polyps that appear in the colon, while epidemiological research suggests that one daily aspirin may cut your risk of digestive tumors by 30 to 50 percent. It is unclear whether one adult aspirin per day or one baby aspirin is enough to do the trick. The other problem, however, is that one aspirin a day could also cause bleeding from the digestive tract. Please consult your physician about this potential tumor buster.

49. Know the Impact
of Environmental Toxins

There are a number of toxins and poisons in our environment that are causing higher rates of cancer. Colon cancer, in particular, has been shown to be much higher in areas where there are hazardous waste sites and widespread pesticide use. Unfortunately, there are far more research dollars being poured into examining hereditary causes of colon cancer than environmental causes. This is odd, considering that roughly 85 percent of colon cancer is considered to be caused spontaneously. Being aware of environmental toxins is the first step in reducing your exposure to them. So what are some known environmental toxins?

Organochlorines are particularly nasty; they're non-degradable in the environment and are fat soluble in the bodies of wildlife and humans. An organochlorine is what you get when you take natural chlorine, found in ordinary salt, and split the salt molecule to make chlorine gas. When that chlorine gas comes into contact with any organic (carbon-based) matter, you wind up with an organochlorine. So organochlorines such as DDT, DDE, dioxins, and PCBs (polychlorinated biphenyls) have accumulated and concentrated in the food chain.

It's estimated that billions of gallons of these toxic substances have been released into an unsuspecting environment. Since these chemicals are resistant to breaking down, they're spread around the world through the air and water, exposing us to these poisons in our food, groundwater, surface water, and air. A 1987 study identified 177 organochlorines in the fat, breast milk, blood, semen, and breath of the general North American population. According to a 1992 Greenpeace report on chlorine and human health, no industrial organochlorines are known to be *non*toxic.

Although PCBs were first introduced into the environment in 1929, large-scale production of man-made chemicals didn't really take place until just after World War II. By 1947, the United States was producing 259,000 pounds of pesticides annually; by 1960, this figure had grown to 636.7 million pounds. For synthetic fibers, between 1945 and 1970 production increased by almost 6,000 percent; plastics production increased by almost 2,000 percent; nitrogen fertilizers and synthetic organic chemicals increased by about 1,000 percent; organic solvents increased by 746 percent.

Industry now produces roughly 40 million tons of chlorine per year. That chlorine is then combined with petrochemicals to make organochlorine products, such as PVC plastic, solvents, pesticides, and refrigerants. After that, thousands of organochlorines occur as by-products—particularly in the pulp and paper industry. These chemicals are spread by wind and water, sprayed on plants, or ingested by animals we eat, and settle in our fat and tissues.

This is a major reason why low-fat diets are related to lower cancer rates. The more fat on your body, the more fat-soluble toxins can be in your body. Organochlorines are associated with higher rates of breast, colon, ovarian, testicular, prostate, and lung cancers.

50. Reduce Exposure to Environmental Toxins

The best way to reduce your exposure to environmental toxins is through the food chain. A heavily criticized 1996 report, released by the Harvard Center for Cancer Prevention, stated that cancer was caused by only four things: tobacco use, diet, obesity, and lack of exercise—all "blame the victim" categories. It attributed only 2 percent of U.S. cancer deaths to "environmental pollution," which it narrowly defined as air pollution and organochlorines. Environmental scientists argue that since the report attributes 30 percent of cancer to diet and obesity, it's crucial that exposures to environmental carcinogens in *food* be counted as "environmental pollutants" rather than simply "diet." For example, the report failed to include drinking water contaminants under "environmental pollution."

The problem with citing "diet" as a cause of cancer, ignoring all the *contaminants* in our diets, is that the Harvard report leaves people with the impression that cancer can be prevented by changing their lifestyles. Although exposure to pollutants and contaminants can occur through your diet, that doesn't mean it's easy to reduce your exposure to air-borne contaminants.

There are similar omissions about environmental hazards in the American Cancer Society's thirty-three-page "Cancer Facts & Figures" booklet, which devotes only two pages to environmental causes of cancer.

Eating organically, and lobbying for more information about what your food was sprayed with, or grown in, or ate, is the best way to eliminate carcinogens from your body. Even though you cannot control the air you breathe, you can still control what you ingest.

So the best place to start the environmental "cleanup" is in your kitchen. Your weekly groceries probably contain residues from pesticides and other organochlorines (on store-bought fruits and vegetables); hormones in meat products, as well as a number of "extras" you may not have bargained for, which were *fed* to your meat sources when they were still alive. These include feed additives, antibiotics, and tranquilizers. Meanwhile, anything packaged most likely contains dyes and flavors from a variety of chemical concoctions.

In addition, when one species becomes unable to reproduce, the food chain is interrupted because it eliminates important food sources that other species depend on for survival. A Native North American saying speaks to this issue: Not until the last river is poisoned, and the last tree cut down, will humans realize that they can't eat money.

Cleaning up the food chain is all part of creating a healthy, contaminant-free diet for ourselves. So make the following grocery list before your next shopping trip:

- You can find out what was fed to your meat sources, and whether they were injected with drugs, by calling the USDA information line at (202) 720-2791.
- You can find out what waters your fish have swum in by calling the number above.
- You can find "safe food" that is organically grown through a number of natural produce supermarkets.
- You can find out what chemicals were sprayed on produce by calling the USDA number above.
- You can find out more about your supermarket's produce buying habits by contacting your supermarket's head office.

Since the origin of the word *consumer* comes from the word *consume*—to eat—becoming vigilantes about our groceries is the only way to help change the produce and foodstuff industry. Customers are incredibly important to every company. In the 1980s, it was the "vigilante consumer" who helped to make manufacturers more environmentally friendly and value conscious. In many instances, the sheer volume of customer complaints and customer letters completely changed not only individual companies' habits and policies, but an entire industry. If enough customers boycott products, protest manufacturing or agricultural practices, and so on, the companies *will* change. Bring new meaning to the adage: The customer is always right!

Worried about the plastic that lines certain canned goods? Demand labeling that identifies the organic chemicals used to *make* that plastic. Worried about the plastics used in various cosmetics, detergents, and spermicides? Then write letters to manufacturers; call 800 numbers; start a newsgroup on the Internet; lobby; protest; boycott products to help change standards. Don't be afraid to write letters to the editor of daily newspapers or call for press conferences on various labeling, packaging, or ingredient issues that concern you. What exactly *is* plastic wrap made out of anyway? *You have a right to know!* What was this spinach *sprayed* with? You have a right to a label that reads: "This produce sprayed with endosulfan."

Epilogue

Think about some of your loved ones who have survived, or perhaps died from colon cancer. If you could have given the information in this book to those people earlier in their lives, it may have spared them a diagnosis of colon cancer. That's because the information in this book may have inspired them to:

- Go for regular screening (numbers 1 through 10).
- Eat fiber and stay regular (numbers 11 through 20).
- Eat less fat (numbers 21 through 30).
- Exercise (numbers 31 through 40).
- Build up the immune system (numbers 41 through 50).

You have in your hands the knowledge you need to prevent colon cancer. But this book provides much more than fifty ways to prevent colon cancer; it gives you fifty ways to prevent unnecessary suffering; fifty ways to prolong your life; and fifty ways to spend more time with your loved ones. Whether you're under thirty-five or over sixty-five, use this information to improve your life, and make your body the best it can be. And when you're finished reading this, be sure to pass it on to someone you think can benefit from these pages.

Good luck and good health!

Glossary

Note: This list is not exhaustive. These are not literal dictionary definitions, but rather definitions created solely for the context of this book. Any resemblance to definitions found in other glossaries or dictionaries is purely coincidental.

adrenaline: a hormone your body secretes that creates "fight-or-flight" symptoms of increased heart rate, sweating, nervousness, dizziness, and so on.

aerobic activity: any activity that causes the heart to pump harder and faster, causing you to breathe faster, which increases the level of oxygen in the bloodstream.

antioxidants: vitamins A, C, and E, and beta-carotene, found in colored (nongreen) fruits and vegetables. Antioxidants prevent the oxidation of cell membranes, which can lead to cancer; they are the cancer-fighting "foot soldiers."

anus: opening from the digestive tract to outside the body; equipped with a muscular sphincter for the expulsion of waste.

barium enema: a chalky solution inserted into the colon, which shows up on x-ray film.

bile: produced by the liver, bile is squeezed out of the gall-bladder (where it is stored between meals) into the bile ducts when you eat, and is used to break down fat into the watery contents of the intestine.

carbohydrates: the building blocks of most foods, which provide energy to the body to fuel the central nervous system; they help the body use vitamins, minerals, amino acids, and other nutrients.

cholesterol: a whitish, waxy fat made in vast quantities by the liver. (*See also* HDL; LDL.)

colon: bottom portion of the digestive tract; a large dehydrator; it extracts all liquid from the waste and turns it into recognizable stool.

colonoscopy: procedure in which a long tube is inserted through the rectum in order to obtain a tissue sample.

colorectal cancer: cancer of the colon and/or rectum.

colorectum: the lining of the tubing in the large intestine; the colorectum is made up mostly of muscle tissue, but contains some fat and lymph tissue.

complex carbohydrates: sophisticated foods made up of larger molecules, such as grain foods and foods high in fiber.

corticosteroids: powerful steroid drugs, such as hydrocortisone and prednisone, that control inflammation and suppress the immune system; they work by mimicking cortisol, an anti-inflammatory hormone made by the adrenal gland.

Crohn's disease: occurs when the inflammation goes beyond the lining into the actual walls of the intestine; also known as ileitis or regional enteritis.

cytokine blockers: the newest edition of drugs added to irritable bowel disorder therapy; researchers have discovered that during a flare-up, cytokines are made, which are proteins that cause inflammation; drugs aimed specifically at these cytokines are a promising new trend in IBD therapy.

digestion: the process by which food is converted into the nutrients we need to live and the excess waste we don't need.

digestive system: a series of tubing, about 22 feet long, that twists and turns from the mouth to the anus.

dysplasia: occurs when the cells that line the colon become precancerous as a result of ulcerative colitis.

fatty acids: crucial nutrients for cells; they also regulate hormone production.

fiber: part of a plant that cannot be digested, which can lower cholesterol levels or improve regularity; also causes a slower rise in glucose levels, which lessens the body's insulin requirements.

fructose: a monosaccharide, or single sugar, that combines with glucose to form sucrose and is one and a half times sweeter than sucrose.

functional foods: foods that have significant levels of biologically active disease-preventing or health promoting properties.

gastroenterologist: a doctor who is a GI (gastrointestinal) specialist.

glucose: a monosaccharide, or single sugar—sugar in its purest form.

HDL: high-density lipoprotein, known as "good" cholesterol.

hemorrhoids: Swollen blood vessels or veins around the anus either inside (internal) or under the skin around it (external).

hydrogenation: process that converts liquid fat to semisolid fat by adding hydrogen.

inflammatory bowel disease (IBD): a serious, chronic condition occurring when one or more parts of the small or large intestine is inflamed, causing symptoms that range from unpleasant but manageable to severe and debilitating.

large intestine: the colon or large bowel; the large intestine stores waste products for a day or two before they are expelled from the body in the form of stools.

LDL: low-density lipoprotein, known as "bad" cholesterol.

nutrients: the by-products created when food and drink are broken down into their smallest parts to provide energy to our cells.

obesity: when you weigh more than 20 percent of your ideal weight for your age and height.

omega-3 fatty acids: naturally present in fish that swim in cold waters; crucial for brain tissue; are all unsaturated, and not only lower cholesterol levels but are said to protect against heart disease.

ostomy: an external pouch placed over the ileum's tip after a proctocolectomy, allowing waste to drain out; combined, these procedures are known as an ileostomy.

phytochemicals: "plant chemicals" (*phyto* is Greek for "plant"); disease-fighting or protective chemicals found in plant foods such as tomatoes, oats, soy, oranges, and broccoli.

polyps: benign tumors in the colon or rectum.

proctocolectomy: the surgery used to treat ulcerative colitis where the entire colon and rectum are removed.

rectum: serves as a holding tank for the stool until it can be expelled from the body.

saturated fat: a fat solid at room temperature (from animal sources) that stimulates the body to produce LDL, or "bad" cholesterol; tropical oils are also saturated even though they are liquid.

sigmoidoscopy: a procedure involving the insertion of a short tube through the rectum with a lighted microscope on its end. Used to obtain a tissue sample.

small intestine: the midgut or small bowel; the small intestine can also be categorized as the duodenum, jejunum, and ileum.

soluble fiber: fiber that is water soluble, or dissolves in water; forms a gel in the body that traps fats and lowers cholesterol.

stomach: an accordionlike bag of muscle and other tissue near the center of the abdomen just below the rib cage; the bag extends to accommodate food and shrinks when it is empty; the stomach itself is a "holding tank" for food until it can be distributed into more distant parts of the gastrointestinal tract.

trans-fatty acids (hydrogenated oils): harmful, man-made fats that not only raise the level of "bad" cholesterol (LDL) in the bloodstream, but lower the amount of "good" cholesterol (HDL) that's already there; produced through the process of hydrogenation.

triglycerides: a combination of saturated, monounsaturated, and polyunsaturated fatty acids and glycerol.

ulcerative colitis: occurs when inflammation and/or ulceration is confined to the inner lining of the colon (colitis) and rectum (proctitis).

unsaturated fat: known as "good fat" because it doesn't cause the body to produce "bad" cholesterol and increases the levels of "good" cholesterol; partially solid or liquid at room temperature.

Bibliography

American Dietetic Association and National Center for Nutrition and Dietetics (NCND). "10 Tips to Healthy Eating" (April 1994).

"Aspirin May Protect Your Colon Against Cancer, Too." *Ladies Home Journal* (March 1998): 131.

Bartlett, J. G. "Epidemiology and Clinical Aspects of Antibiotic-Associated Colitis." Proceedings of the 2nd International Symposium on Anaerobes, June 22, 1985, Tokyo, Japan.

Bayer Healthcare Division. "Exercise: Guidelines to a Healthier You." Patient information (1997).

———. "Food and Exercise: Guidelines to a Healthier You." Patient information (1997).

Berndl, Leslie, R.D., M.Sc. "Understanding Fat." *Diabetes Dialogue* 42, no. 1 (Spring 1995).

Beyers, Joanne, R.D. "How Sweet It Is!" *Diabetes Dialogue* 42, no. 1 (Spring 1995).

Bondy, M., and C. Mastromarino. "Ethical Issues of Genetic Testing and Their Implications in Epidemiologic Studies." *Annals of Epidemiology* 7 (July 1997): 363–66.

Boston University Medical Center. "Constipation: Causes." Booklet (1996).

Bove, C. M., et al. "Presymptomatic and Predisposition Genetic Testing: Ethical and Social Considerations. *Seminars in Oncology Nursing* (May 13, 1997): 135–40.

Britt, Beverley. "Pesticides and Alternatives." Excerpted from the Canadian Organic Growers Toronto Chapter's Spring Conference, pp. 1–4.

"A Cancer Gene Makes Colon Removal an Option." *New York Times* (March 19, 1997).

Caplan, L. S. "Disparities in Breast Cancer Screening: Is It Ethical?" *Public Health Review* 25 (1997): 31–41.

CCFA National Scientific Advisory Committee, Division of Digestive Diseases, University of North Carolina, Chapel Hill. 1997 Research Report. Posted to: MedicineNet, Information Network, Inc. www.medicinenet.com.

Chaddock, Brenda, C.D.E. "Activity Is Key to Diabetes Health." *Canadian Pharmacy Journal* (March 1997): 14.

———. "Foul Weather Fitness: The Hardest Part Is Getting Started." *Canadian Pharmacy Journal* (March 1996): 42.

———. "The Magic of Exercise." *Canadian Pharmacy Journal* (September 1995): 45.

"Chemical in Green Tea Stops Tumors, Study Says." Reuters (June 5, 1998).

Christrup, Janet. "Nuts About Nuts: The Joys of Growing Nut Trees." *Cognition* (July 1991): 20–22.

Clarke, Bill. "Action Figures." *Diabetes Dialogue* 43, no. 3 (Fall 1996).

Colborn, Theo, John Peterson Myers, and Dianne Dumanoski. *Our Stolen Future*. New York: Dutton, 1996.

"Combat Job Stress: Does Work Make You Sick?" Retrieved online: http://www.convoke.com/ markjr/cjstress.html (February 12, 1999).

"Crohn's Disease and Colitis." Crohn's and Colitis Foundation of Canada (1995).

Cronier, Claire, M.Sc., R.D. "Sweetest Choices." *Diabetes Dialogue* 44, no. 1 (Spring 1997).

Cunningham, John J., Ph.D., F.A.C.N. "Vitamins, Minerals, and Diabetes." Excerpted from Canadian Diabetes Association Conference, 1995.

Dashe, Alfred M., M.D. *The Man's Health Sourcebook*, 2d ed. Los Angeles: Lowell House, 1999.

Dickens, Bernard M., Nancy Pei, and Kathryn M. Taylor. "Legal and Ethical Issues in Genetic Testing and Counseling for Susceptibility to Breast, Ovarian and Colon Cancer." *Canadian Medical Association Journal* 154, no. 6 (March 15, 1996): 813–18.

Drum, David, and Terry Zierenberg. *The Type 2 Diabetes Sourcebook*, 2d ed. Los Angeles: Lowell House, 2000.

Engel, June V., Ph.D., "Beyond Vitamins: Phytochemicals to Help Fight Disease." *Health News* 14, University of Toronto (June 1996).

———. "Eating Fibre." *Diabetes Dialogue* 44, no. 1 (Spring 1997).

"Engineering a Treatment for Crohn's Disease." *The Lancet* 349, no. 9051 (February 1997).

"Everyday Carcinogens: Stopping Cancer Before It Starts." Proceedings from the March 1999 Workshop on Primary Cancer Prevention, McMaster University, Hamilton, Ontario, Canada.

Farquhar, Andrew, M.D. "Exercising Essentials." *Diabetes Dialogue* 43, no. 3 (Fall 1996): 6–8.

Feldman, Gayle. "Is Genetic Testing Right for You?" *Self* (October 1996): 187–209.

Food and Drug Administration. "Nutrient Claims Guide for Individual Foods." Special Report, Focus on Food Labeling. FDA Publication No. 95-2289.

Fraser, Eliabeth, R.D., C.D.E., and Bill Clarke. "Loafing Around." *Diabetes Dialogue* 44, no. 1 (Spring 1997).

Gabrys, Jennifer, B.Sc.Pharm., C.D.E. "Ask the Professionals." *Diabetes Dialogue* 43, no. 4 (Winter 1996).

Gilbert, Susan. "Doctors Often Misread Results of Genetic Tests, Study Finds." *New York Times* (March 26, 1997).

Gordon, Dennis. "Acarbose: When It Works/When It Doesn't." *Diabetes Forecast* (February 1997).

Harries, A. D., V. A. Danis, and R. V. Heatley. "Influence of Nutritional Status on Immune Functions in Patients with Crohn's Disease." *Gut* 25 (1984): 465–72.

Harrison, Pam. "Rethinking Obesity." *Family Practice* 13, no. 2 (March 11, 1996).

Healy, Bernadette, M.D. "BRCA Genes—Bookmaking, Fortunetelling, and Medical Care." *The New England Journal of Medicine* 336, no. 20 (May 15, 1997): 1448–49.

"The Heart Healthy Kitchen." *Countdown USA: Countdown to a Healthy Heart.* Published by Allegheny General Hospital and Voluntary Hospitals of America, Inc., 1990.

Hendler, Saul Sheldon, M.D., Ph.D. *The Doctors' Vitamin and Mineral Encyclopedia.* New York: Fireside Books, 1990.

Hilts, Philip. "Risks of Colon Cancer." *New York Times* (April 24, 1997).

Hislop, Gregory T., M.D.C.M., "The Role of Nutrition in the Prevention of Cancer." *The Canadian Journal of CME* (March 1995): 111–18.

Ho, Marian, MSc., R.D. "Learning Your ABCs, Part Two." *Diabetes Dialogue* 43, no. 3 (Fall 1996).

Hoffman-La Roche, Ltd. "The Antioxidant Connection: Visiting Speakers Discuss Immunity, Diabetes." Published by the Vitamin Information Program of Hoffman-La Roche, Ltd. (September 1995).

"How to Deal with Stress," Retrieved online from: http://www.backrelief.com/stress.htm (February 12, 1999).

Hunt, John A., M.B., F.R.C.P.C. "Fueling Up." *Diabetes Dialogue* 41, no. 4 (Winter 1994).

Hunter, J. E., and T. H. Applewhite. "Reassessment of Trans-fatty Acid Availability in the U.S. Diet." *American Journal of Clinical Nutrition* 54 (1991): 363–69.

Hurley, Jane, and Stephen Schmidt. "Going with the Grain." *Nutrition Action* (October 1994): 10–11.

International Food Information Council. "Antibiotics in Animals: An Interview with Stephen Sundlof, D.V.M., Ph.D." *IFIC Review*, 1100 Connecticut Avenue NW, Suite 430, Washington, DC 20036 (1997).

———. "Intense Sweeteners: Effects on Appetite and Weight Management." *IFIC Review*, 1100 Connecticut Avenue NW, Suite 430, Washington, DC 20036 (November 1995).

———. "Putting Fun Back into Food," *IFIC Review*, 1100 Connecticut Avenue NW, Suite 430, Washington, DC 20036 (1997).

———. "Q&A About Fatty Acids and Dietary Fats." *IFIC Review*, 1100 Connecticut Avenue NW, Suite 430, Washington, DC 20036 (1997).

———. "Sorting Out the Facts About Fat." *IFIC Review*, 1100 Connecticut Avenue NW, Suite 430, Washington, DC 20036 (1997).

———. "Uses and Nutritional Impact of Fat Reduction Ingredients." *IFIC Review*, 1100 Connecticut Avenue NW, Suite 430, Washington, DC 20036 (October 1995).

———. "What You Should Know About Aspartame." *IFIC Review*, 1100 Connecticut Avenue NW, Suite 430, Washington, DC 20036 (November 4, 1996).

———. "What You Should Know About Sugars." *IFIC Review,* 1100 Connecticut Avenue NW, Suite 430, Washington, DC 20036 (May 1994).

International Joint Commission. "Eighth Biennial Report on Great Lakes Water Quality, Under the Great Lakes Water Quality Agreement of 1978 to the Governments of the United States and Canada and the State and Provincial Governments of the Great Lakes Basin." International Joint Commission, 1250 23rd Street NW, Suite 100, Washington, DC 20440 (1996).

Ionescu, Simona-Adriana, M.D. "Causes of Breast and Colon Cancer in Romania." Paper presented at the World Conference on Breast Cancer, July 13–17, 1997, Kingston, Ontario, Canada.

Kea, David. "Herd Health: The Biggest Reward of Ecological Dairy Farming." *Cognition* 93 (Winter 1992): 26–27.

Kishi, Misa, M.D. "Impact of Pesticides on Health in Developing Countries: Research, Policy and Actions." Paper presented at the World Conference on Breast Cancer, July 13–17, 1997, Kingston, Ontario, Canada.

Kock, Henry. "Restoring Natural Vegetation as Part of the Farm." *Gardening Without Chemicals '91,* Canadian Organic Growers Toronto Chapter (April 6, 1991).

Kuczmarski, R. J., K. M. Flegal, S. M. Campbell, and C. L. Johnson. "Increasing Prevalence of Overweight Among U.S. Adults: The National Health and Nutrition Examination Surveys, 1960 to 1991." *Journal of the American Medical Association* 272, no. 3 (July 1994): 205–11.

Kushi, Michio. *The Cancer Prevention Guide.* New York: St. Martin's Press, 1993.

Lembo, Anthony (ed.). "IBS and Crohn's-Colitis FAQ." Posted to: alt.support.crohns-colitis *and* alt.support.ibs. (E-mail queries to alembo@UCLA.edu or juniper@uiuc.edu.)

Liebman, Bonnie. "Walking and Cancer." *Nutrition Action* (March 1998): 13.

McAuliffe, Kathleen, "Dying of Embarrassment." *More* (May/June 1999): 52–62.

National Institute of Diabetes and Digestive and Kidney Diseases. "Ulcerative Colitis." NIH Publication No. 95-1597 (April 1992).

"Oats Are In." *Countdown USA: Countdown to a Healthy Heart.* Published by Allegheny General Hospital and Voluntary Hospitals of America, Inc., 1990.

"Olestra: Yes or No?" Excerpted from the *University of California at Berkeley Wellness Letter,* in *Diabetes Dialogue* 43, no. 3 (Fall 1996).

Ontario Breast Cancer Information Exchange Project. "A Guide to Unconventional Cancer Therapies." Booklet (1994).

Parens, Erik. "Glad and Terrified: On the Ethics of BRCA1 and 2 Testing." *Cancer Investigation* 14, no. 4 (1996): 405–11.

"Patient Information." The National Digestive Diseases Information Clearinghouse (NDDIC), a service of the National Institute of Diabetes and Digestive and Kidney Diseases, part of the National Institutes of Health, under the U.S. Public Health Service.

National Digestive Diseases Information Clearinghouse, Licensed to Medical Strategies, Inc. (1996).

"Physical Activity." *Equilibrium.* Canadian Diabetes Association no. 1 (1996).

"Position of the American Dietetic Association: Use of Nutritive and Nonnutritive Sweeteners." *Journal of the American Dietetic Association* 93 (1993): 816–22.

PROSWEET Canada. "Choosing Your Sweetener." Product information (1997).

———. "The Low-Calorie Pure Sugar Taste Sweetener." Product information (1997).

"Q&A on Low-Calorie Sweeteners." *The Diabetes News* 1, no. 2 (Spring 1997).

Reilly, P. R., et al. "Ethical Issues in Genetic Research: Disclosure and Informed Consent." *Nature and Genetics* 15 (January 15, 1997): 16–20.

"Return of Crohn's." *The Lancet* 349, no. 9053 (March 1997).

Rifkin, Jeremy. "Playing God with the Genetic Code." *Health Naturally* (April/May 1995): 40–44.

Rosenthal, M. Sara. *The Breast Sourcebook*, 2d. ed. Los Angeles: Lowell House, 1999.

———. *The Breastfeeding Sourcebook*, 2d. ed. Los Angeles: Lowell House, 1998.

———. *The Gastrointestinal Sourcebook*. Los Angeles: Lowell House, 1999.

———. *The Pregnancy Sourcebook*, 3d. ed. Los Angeles: Lowell House, 1999.

————. *The Thyroid Sourcebook*, 3d. ed. Los Angeles: Lowell House, 1998.

————. *The Type 2 Diabetic Woman*. Los Angeles: Lowell House, 1999.

Rudd, Wm. Warren. *Advice from the Rudd Clinic: A Guide to Colorectal Health*. Toronto: Macmillan Canada, 1997.

Seto, Carol, R.D., C.D.E. "Nutrition Labeling—U.S. Style." *Diabetes Dialogue* 42, no. 1 (Spring 1995).

Shimer, Porter. *Keeping Fitness Simple: 500 Tips for Fitting Exercise into Your Life*. Pownal, Vt.: Storey Books, 1998.

Slattery, Mary L., et al. "Dietary Energy Sources and Colon Cancer Risk." *American Journal of Epidemiology* 145 (1997): 199–210.

Soto, Ana M., Honorata Justicia, Jonathan W. Wray, and Carlos Sonnenschein. "*p*-Nonyl-Phenol: An Estrogenic Xenobiotic Released from 'Modified' Polystyrene." *Environmental Health Perspectives* 92 (1991): 167–73.

Splenda Information Centre. "Sucralose Overview." Product information (1997).

Sponselli, Christina. "Genetic Testing Raises Questions." *Nurseweek* (November 1997).

————. "RNs Can Answer Questions About Genetics." *Nurseweek* (November 1997).

Stehlin, Dori. "A Little Lite Reading." Posted to FDA Web site: http://www.fda.gov/fdac/foodlabel/diabetes.html. (Retrieved January 11, 1999.)

Steingraber, Sandra. *Living Downstream: An Ecologist Looks at Cancer and the Environment.* New York: Addison-Wesley, 1997.

Stone, D. H., and S. Stewart. "Screening and the New Genetics; A Public Health Perspective on the Ethical Debate." *Journal of Public Health Medicine* 18 (March 1996): 3–5.

"Stress." Retrieved online from: http://meagherlab.tamu.edu/ M-Meagher/Abnormal/stressout (February 12, 1999).

Vegetarian Resource Group. *Getting to the Roots of a Vegetarian Diet.* Baltimore, Md.: Vegetarian Resource Group, 1997.

Willett, W. C., et al. "Intake of Trans-fatty Acids and Risk of Coronary Heart Disease Among Women." *The Lancet* 341: 581–85 (1993).

Wormworth, Janice. "Toxins and Tradition: The Impact of Food-Chain Contamination on the Inuit of Northern Quebec." *Canadian Medical Association Journal* 152, no. 8 (April 15, 1995).

Index

A

active living, 59–60
additives, food, 51, 82
adrenaline, 87
aerobic activity, definition
   of, 59–60, 87
aerobic exercise, 56–58
air pollution, 81
anemia, 13
animal fat, 45, 49
anoscope exam, 6
anticancer agents, 69, 70,
   77–79
antioxidants, 69, 70, 87
anus, 87
aspirin, 79
Ayurvedic medicine, 29

B

barium enema, 8–9, 88
benign tumors. *See* polyps
beta-carotene, 70
bile, 88
biopsies, 10, 12
blood sugar. *See* glucose
blood tests, 6–7, 13
Borg scale, 58–59
bowel movements
   colon training, 31
   fiber and, 19–20
   hemorrhoids, 27
   "lazy bowel," 30
   modifying your diet, 28
   normal, 24–25
   understanding laxatives,
      29–30
   urgent, 11–12